More praise for *Carville's Cure*

"By turns heart-wrenching, inspiring, and infuriating, this is a fast-paced and highly readable account of attempts by patients, their families, doctors, and American society in general to deal with the world's most misunderstood disease. Written with the eye of an experienced journalist and the voice of a novelist, this book tells the story—stranger than fiction—of the patients, nuns, doctors, movie stars, and politicians who have struggled to come to terms with the stigma and discrimination attached to leprosy. The book is painstakingly researched and documented, and unfolds dramatically through the words of the patients and other participants through their letters and personal papers as well as newspaper accounts and interviews."

—David Scollard, retired director, National
Hansen's Disease Program

"[A] fine history, by turns heartbreaking and infuriating. . . . A caustic story told with empathy and a sharp eye for society's intolerance."

—*Kirkus Reviews*

"Polished and compassionate. . . . [Pam Fessler's] well-researched and articulate account humanizes sufferers and caregivers alike, and offers hope in the medical field's ability to halt the spread of contagious illness. Readers will be enlightened and encouraged."

—*Publishers Weekly*

"Heartbreaking and infuriating."

—Tony Miksanek, *Booklist*

CARVILLE'S CURE

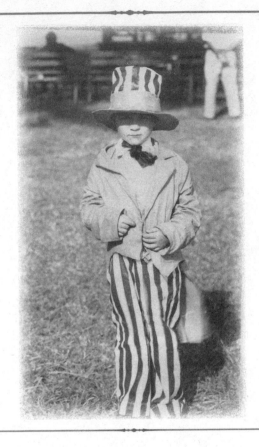

A young Carville patient at a Fourth of July celebration.

CARVILLE'S CURE

Leprosy, Stigma, and the Fight for Justice

PAM FESSLER

LIVERIGHT PUBLISHING CORPORATION
A Division of W. W. Norton & Company
Independent Publishers Since 1923

Frontispiece credit: Courtesy, Daughters of Charity
Province of St. Louise, St. Louis, MO.

For information about permission to reproduce selections from this book, write to
Permissions, Liveright Publishing Corporation, a division of
W. W. Norton & Company, Inc., 500 Fifth Avenue, New York, NY 10110

For information about special discounts for bulk purchases, please contact
W. W. Norton Special Sales at specialsales@wwnorton.com or 800-233-4830

Manufacturing by Lake Book Manufacturing
Book design by Patrice Sheridan
Production manager: Julia Druskin

ISBN 978-1-63149-503-8

Liveright Publishing Corporation, 500 Fifth Avenue, New York, N.Y. 10110
www.wwnorton.com

W. W. Norton & Company Ltd., 15 Carlisle Street, London W1D 3BS

1 2 3 4 5 6 7 8 9 0

For David and Peter

Mercy is no substitute for justice.

—Sister Catherine Sullivan

Contents

Author's Note

I HAVE AVOIDED using the word *leper* to describe individuals with Hansen's disease except in quotes or when it is unavoidable, as in referring to the Louisiana Leper Home. I have used *leprosy* more frequently, and interchangeably with *Hansen's disease*, because it is the term still commonly used in many parts of the world.

CARVILLE'S CURE

Prologue

IT WAS ALMOST nighttime when the rain began to fall in torrents, rushing down the side of the hill that Morris Kolnitzky and several hundred other American soldiers had fought so hard to climb. They were exhausted as they rested not far from Fort Pandapatan, on the southern Philippine island of Mindanao. Muslim rebels were holed up inside, determined to drive back the Americans. The infantrymen had been under fire all afternoon, caught between the shells launched from U.S. artillery mountain guns behind them and bullets pouring down from the fort above.[1]

The soldiers had come within yards of the fort only to find it surrounded by ditches filled with sharpened bamboo stakes and by rebels wielding short, double-edged swords. The infantrymen fought back with their guns and bayonets, but within minutes dozens of men on both sides had been killed or injured. As the sun set, and the rain and fog rolled in, the Americans were ordered to retreat and to pull their wounded comrades to safety.

It was May 2, 1902, and Kolnitzky had arrived in the Philippines only a few weeks earlier, along with the other young men of the 27th Infantry. They were fresh recruits, brought in to quash an insurrection that had erupted at the end of the Spanish-American War. The soldiers had barely had time to adjust to the oppressive tropical heat and thick jungle terrain, let alone to the violence of battle. Kolnitzky was among the youngest, only seventeen years old. Lying there in the mud and the dark, hearing the cries of the injured men, he must have been terrified, knowing how easily a bullet or the thrust of a sword could end his short life.

What Kolnitzky did not know, as he waited in a flooded trench, was that he faced another, more insidious threat, one that no gun or bayonet could stop. And one that would eventually take his life. A tiny rod-shaped germ, *Mycobacterium leprae*, would enter his body, possibly there in the mud, or later as he camped in close quarters with someone who was already infected. The germ would quietly stew in Kolnitzky's body for years, duplicating at an extraordinarily slow pace, as he went on to start a business and raise a family back home in America. Over time, it would attack his peripheral nerves, causing numbness in his fingers and toes. It would turn his hands into claws and rob him of his eyesight. It would force him to flee from his home in the middle of the night to avoid being incarcerated for life.

———

As the 27th Infantry fought its way across the Philippines, a small band of nuns waged another battle halfway around the world. Their commander was the formidable Sister Benedicta Roach, one of four Daughters of Charity trying desperately to care for more than three dozen patients at the Louisiana Leper Home. The home was located on an old sugar plantation seventy miles up the Mississippi River from New Orleans, on an isolated strip of land that jutted into the river like an upside-down thumb.

The patients and sisters had been all but abandoned there. The plantation grounds were muddy and overgrown, and the housing—former slave cabins for the patients, an old mansion for the sisters—was dilapidated. The Louisiana air was so thick and humid you could grab it in your hands. Sister Benedicta knew that their biggest challenge was not leprosy but the mosquitoes that flourished around them and an unpredictable water supply. A few months earlier, her predecessor, Sister Beatrice Hart, had died from malaria and exhaustion.

In the spring of 1902 conditions were only getting worse, and Sister Benedicta decided to go to New Orleans to confront members of the Louisiana Leper Home Board of Control in person. The men balked at her request for more funds, but she would not back down. "Gentleman, I shall be at St. Vincent's Infant Asylum until four o'clock this afternoon," she told them. "If at that hour I have not heard from you, I shall make public appeal through the newspapers. The people of New Orleans will not tolerate having the sisters care for the lepers without even water to keep them clean."[2]

Her ultimatum worked. Money was approved for a water plant and for the construction of new cottages for the patients. It was a decisive moment for a home that would eventually become one of the leading leprosaria in the world, where thousands of Americans would be confined—with both miraculous and tragic results.

Among those who would end up there was Morris Kolnitzky, who spent years in New York concealing his disease, as he fought both its debilitating symptoms and centuries of superstition. His teenage son would come home from school one day to find that his father was gone, taken away by public health officials and isolated, not out of medical necessity but from ignorance and fear. Kolnitzky's son was my father-in-law. He never saw or spoke to his father again and, because of the stigma and shame, kept his father's illness a secret for more than sixty years.

————

This is the story of the thousands of patients, families, and caregivers in the United States who struggled against one of the world's most dreaded and misunderstood diseases. Their enemy was a physical illness, but also a social one. In many ways, the stigma of leprosy was far worse than the disease itself. It would prove far more difficult to cure.

The irony is that leprosy, now called Hansen's disease, is one of the least contagious diseases. The overwhelming majority of human beings—95 percent—are naturally immune, and for those who are not, leprosy is extremely difficult to contract. Scientists still don't know exactly how the disease spreads, but they do know that it requires prolonged, close contact with the germ. Not one medical worker or staff member at the Louisiana leprosarium, which eventually became known as Carville, became infected in more than a hundred years of operation. While victims can suffer loss of sensation in their hands and feet, leading to crippled limbs and amputation, the disease does not cause skin and fingers to fall off, as many people believe. Some patients go blind or suffer from painful lesions and disfigurement, but many have few obvious symptoms at all.

The truth is that for centuries tens of millions of people around the world have been unnecessarily scorned, isolated, and imprisoned. Fear of leprosy has been largely fear of the unknown, inflamed by biblical depictions of the disease as God's way of punishing sinners by condemning them to a life of suffering and scorn. The Old Testament instructed that the afflicted be banished and cry "Unclean, unclean!" to warn others to stay away. But in a cruel and unfortunate twist, what was called leprosy in the Bible was almost certainly not that at all, but an assortment of other skin ailments. Still, the myths and misunderstanding persisted, trailing victims down medieval streets, through the pages of literature, into modern-day life. They justified prejudice against immigrants and others whom society feared. Worse, they hindered treatment for what was a painful and disabling disease, and limited efforts to find a cure.

During the twentieth century, leprosy patients went to Carville to be cared for and, more often than not, isolated for life. Some arrived voluntarily because they were seriously ill and had nowhere else to go. But many were taken there against their will, sometimes in shackles or locked in the boxcars of trains. One man came in the back of a hearse. Another was hidden in a bag.[3] Patients were torn from their families, and babies born inside Carville were taken from their mothers and put up for adoption. Parents abandoned children; husbands abandoned wives.

Those confined to the leprosarium lost not only their freedom but their identity and their civil rights. Until 1946, patients were stripped of their right to vote. In the eyes of the law they were seen more as inmates than as the innocent victims of a serious disease. New arrivals were advised to assume aliases to protect their families from embarrassment and attack. Morris Kolnitzky, who shortened his name after the war to Koll, became Morris Krug. In Carville's cemetery, tombstones were more likely to bear a patient's alias and case number than his or her actual name. For more than a century, this was a world unto itself and unlike any other.

Yet Carville turned out to be as much a refuge as it was a prison for those who lived there. In some ways, patients were more liberated inside the fenced-in grounds, living among others with the same disease, than they were on the outside. This was a place where they could find solace and fellowship, even love, where people did not cringe at the mere mention of the word *leprosy*. Many Carville patients persevered, carving out meaningful, happy lives behind the fences and walls that separated them from the rest of the world. They were a smorgasbord of Americans—a butcher from New York, a debutante from New Orleans, farmworkers from Texas, a Talmudic scholar from Pennsylvania. They were social outcasts, but inside Carville they created their own diverse, vibrant community, with theater and sports teams, Mardi Gras parades and a crusading newspaper. In the Jim Crow South, they had an integrated classroom. Blacks and whites, Hispanics and Asians mixed with an ease that was not seen in the rest of the country for decades.

Over time, the leprosarium also became a kind of incubator, for medical workers desperately seeking a cure and for patients trying to convince a skeptical world they were not the threat many people believed them to be. Those stuck inside Carville reflected American optimism, confident that one day they might be free to go on with their lives. The patients became leading advocates for victims of leprosy and fought to eliminate use of the word *leper* as a synonym for that which is despised and to be avoided at all costs.

The Carville leprosarium was established with the hope that isolating patients would eventually eliminate the disease. Instead, it allowed society to forget they were there. It's a common reaction to that which we fear and don't understand, whether it's leprosy, mental illness, addiction, disability, or AIDS. Isolate and ignore the problem; maybe it will just go away. We seem destined to repeat the mistake. Such actions are easiest when the victims are vilified, and seldom has that been more true than for those with leprosy. They became the ultimate "other"—social outcasts to be blamed for society's ills.[4] Such disdain continues to this day, in a world where hundreds of thousands of new Hansen's disease cases are diagnosed each year.

My father-in-law, Harold Koll, was fifteen years old when his father was taken away in 1935. The impact was devastating, with both the loss of a loved one and the burden of secrecy. Harold's mother made him and his siblings promise to never tell anyone that their father had leprosy, or, she warned, it would ruin the family. Harold was seventy-eight years old when he finally revealed the truth, inspired by a niece who disclosed that she had been sexually abused as a child. He saw how secrets could corrode a life.[5]

Even then, in 1998, my father-in-law knew almost nothing about Hansen's disease or where his father had gone. We eventually discovered the existence of Carville and took him there to see where Morris had spent the final three years of his life and to visit his gravesite in a small Jewish cemetery in nearby Baton Rouge. We found Morris's tombstone in a far corner, standing tilted and alone like an afterthought. Even in death, the leprosy patient was isolated and forgotten. Harold placed a small stack of twigs on top of the marble headstone to show that he had finally come to pay his respects. It was heartbreaking to watch an elderly man discover after all these years what had become of his father and so many others. And to learn that his story was hardly the only one.

Chapter 1

Exile

CLARA MERTZ ARRIVED in New Orleans in February of 1893, locked in a Southern Pacific boxcar and listed as "freight" on the bill of lading. When she got there, the train car was quickly emptied and disinfected, and the young woman was loaded into a carriage to be taken to the city's pesthouse on Hagan Avenue. The pesthouse was really just a collection of decaying wooden shacks, located on a muddy piece of land on the outskirts of town and surrounded by rotting trash. Everything was done with the utmost secrecy, for if word got out about the new arrival, it would be disastrous for the railroad. Only a few officials with the Southern Pacific knew the truth about their cargo, that the twenty-two-year-old woman had leprosy.

Mertz had been sick for years, but she was so ill now, her body covered in painful sores, that her impoverished parents could no longer care for her. They had little choice but to send their daughter, like a sack of rice, across 130 miles of flat, swampy terrain from their home in New Iberia, Louisiana, to New Orleans. The city at least had hospitals and doctors and offered some hope for survival. At that point, Mertz had little left to lose. She came to the city with one dress, a few undergarments, and a very uncertain fate.[1]

The young woman happened to arrive on Fat Tuesday, as the streets of New Orleans were filling with masked Mardi Gras revelers, who danced and drank, seemingly without a care. She must have despaired knowing that this fanciful world would never be hers. The raucous crowds cheered as floats passed by in the annual tribute to fantasy and excess. One carried fairies under a crown of butterflies and roses, surrounded by silver-clad creatures called the "messengers of joy and content." Another bore the Carnival King on a jewel-studded throne beneath a canopy of vines.[2] At the head of the parade was the sacrificial "boeuf gras," a fattened bull with a garland of roses around its neck. It was a sign of the impending arrival of Lent and a harbinger of worse things to come.

Despite the frivolity, these were anxious times. The nearby waterfront was hectic, but deceptively so. Bales of cotton and barrels of sugar and molasses sat stacked on the levees, waiting to be shipped north and abroad. The Mississippi River was like a city itself, with ships urgently squeezing past one another, sending thick smoke into the air. But by 1893 the docks were not nearly as busy as they used to be. New Orleans had once been the second largest port in the country, the fourth largest in the world. Now, it faced stiff competition from Midwest railroads and Hawaiian sugar producers. High wharf fees, crime, labor disputes, and civil unrest encouraged shippers to look elsewhere. Two years earlier, an angry mob had stormed the city jail, shooting and lynching eleven Italians after they were acquitted of murdering the police chief. The violence was encouraged by none other than the mayor, Joseph Shakspeare, who called the thousands of Italian immigrants who had come to the city looking for work "filthy" and "worthless."[3]

Port traffic was down for another, more ominous, reason. The damp, mosquito-ridden city was known as a "pest-hole" and the unhealthiest place in the country. When Mertz arrived, New Orleans had no sewage system, trash collection, or water-treatment plant. Garbage was dumped right into the river. Foul-smelling water pooled in the streets. As uncomfortable as it could be for humans, the tropical climate made the city a paradise for insects and disease. A yellow fever epidemic in 1878 had killed more than 4,400 New Orleanians, most of them children. Then smallpox killed 1,200 more. Neighboring states threatened to tear up railroad tracks and shoot at boats from the city in an effort to avoid a similar fate. New Orleanians called their town the Crescent City, but others called it the "necropolis."[4]

As the Mardi Gras festivities got into full swing, residents were understandably worried about what new threats awaited, hidden in shipments of imported coffee and fruit and among the thousands of immigrants pouring in from abroad. There were germs and diseases everywhere that could wreak havoc on an unprepared city, and more seemed to be emerging each day. Leprosy was the latest to fear.[5]

The city's main newspapers fueled the unease, especially the *Daily Picayune*. It warned readers that an Italian fruit-stand vendor and a woman running a grocery store on North Peters Street both showed signs of leprosy but were still allowed to handle customers' food. The paper complained that "lepers" mingled freely in crowds, endangering public health, and that no official was raising an alarm. The *Picayune* demanded that the city do something to isolate those who had the "loathsome" disease, or at least place warning flags outside their homes. Dr. Joseph C. Beard, who ran the pesthouse where Mertz was taken, falsely claimed that New Orleans was "the only city in the world where lepers were allowed perfect freedom and could walk the streets without restraint."[6]

The *Picayune* employee who covered the story with exceptional zeal was an eighteen-year-old cub reporter named John Smith Kendall. Like all newcomers to the paper, Kendall was assigned one of its most tedious beats, covering the Board of Health. His job was to compile a list of the latest births, marriages, and deaths for a column called Vital Statistics. It was mind-numbing work, but Kendall was inquisitive and ambitious and soon noticed that a curious cause of death—leprosy—was listed with surprising frequency. Like a good reporter, he decided to follow up by visiting the victims' families to learn more. What he quickly learned was that people did not want to talk about it. One outraged widow chased him out of her house. Others denied that their loved ones had ever had the disease. No one wanted to hear such news, but Kendall reported it anyway. Dr. Beard told him there were two people living with leprosy on Franklin Street and another one on Common. Kendall soon became known as the newspaper's "leper" reporter.

A day or two after Mertz's arrival, Kendall was sitting in the *Picayune's* downtown office reading a book. "It was one of those quiet, hot, sleepy afternoons when, in New Orleans nobody expects anything to happen and when as a rule nothing does happen," he later recalled.[7] Another reporter sat at a nearby desk typing a story. The two men were so engrossed, they barely noticed when a shabbily dressed visitor entered the room and took a drink of water from a tank in the corner, using a communal cup. He then walked over to Kendall's colleague, sat down, and announced, "I'm a leper." The startled reporter immediately jumped up and away from the visitor. "Don't you dare touch my desk! That's your man!" he said, pointing to Kendall. "Don't come near me!"[8] The stranger then turned to Kendall and told his story. He lived in Dr. Beard's pesthouse with six other leprosy patients, including a young woman who had just arrived from New Iberia. The pesthouse was where the city was supposed to be caring for those with contagious diseases. The man invited Kendall to come see for himself how they were really being treated.

The young reporter was eager to do so. With his fair hair neatly combed to the side, his jacket buttoned close to his neck, Kendall looked more like a choirboy than a muckraking journalist. But he knew a good story when he saw one. He was also sympathetic to the plight of the "unfortunates," as leprosy patients were frequently called at the time.

A few days later, Kendall hopped on his bicycle and rode to the pesthouse at the edge of the city. He was shocked to see that it was nothing like the asylum he had imagined. Instead, Kendall found a "cluster of miserable and dilapidated buildings above whose portals might be written the significant and fateful words, 'Ye who enter here leave all hope behind.'" He said the conditions were unfit "for cattle or dogs." The courtyard was filled with trash and the kitchen emitted a nauseating odor. Inside, the rooms were damp and gloomy, with "dirty, foul-smelling walls that echo back all day the sobs and moans of the dying lepers, the fateful cry that echoed through the streets of Jerusalem, 'Unclean, unclean, unclean.'"

The young man was admittedly frightened. "To stand within the portals of a leper land is enough to make the hero who could face the cannon's mouth, pause and consider," he wrote later that week. "The second sensation, however, is a feeling of pity and of sorrow, a desire to face the danger in order to better the lot of these people, dying the slow torturing death of the leper, shut out from all humanity, and reaping the curse of an hereditary sin for which they are not responsible."[9]

Inside the pesthouse, Kendall found the young woman from New Iberia sitting alone in a dark room, crying by the window, her mouth twitching between sobs. "The face is a horrid mass of diseased flesh, her body covered with sores, her eyes are blinded with putrid matter," he reported. "Day by day pieces of flesh are dropping from her and whatever she was once, whatever of grace or loveliness she possessed in common with her sex, naught is left."

Mertz's flesh almost certainly was not dropping off and Kendall mistakenly called her Clara "Matts." But no matter, he had a sensational scoop. The seven patients at the pesthouse were supposed to be in the care of Dr. Beard, who was paid twenty-five dollars a month by the city for each person he allegedly treated.[10] But Beard was nowhere in sight. The patients told Kendall that it would sometimes be months between the doctor's visits. They tried to manage on their own with limited medicine and supplies, bandaging each other's wounds and preparing their meals with whatever food they could find. Frequently, there was little food at all.[11]

Picayune readers were incensed, by both the inhumane treatment of the patients and the city's apparent neglect of the public's health. Residents demanded that local officials investigate the contract with Dr. Beard and also do something to stop the disease from spreading. Leprosy had been around Louisiana for more than a hundred years—widely believed to have arrived with West Indian slaves and Acadians from Nova Scotia, although no one was sure—but more cases appeared to be popping up each day.[12] The *New Orleans Medical and Surgical Journal* reported that Charity Hospital alone had treated forty-two cases over a five-year period, while earlier reports had identified only a handful of patients in the entire state. Still, leprosy was notoriously difficult to diagnose and was easily confused with more common illnesses such as syphilis. It was unclear whether the disease was actually spreading or whether more people were simply looking for signs of it.[13]

Growing hysteria and xenophobia made reality irrelevant. By the late 1800s, there were fears of a leprosy pandemic, fueled by rampant anti-immigrant rhetoric and a growing awareness of the power of germs. Asian immigrants, already a target for those who believed they were taking Americans' jobs, were especially suspect. Denis Kearney, a labor leader and racist firebrand, traveled the country railing against "moon-eyed lepers"—at one point parading a Chinese man disfigured by the disease through the streets of San Francisco to make his case.[14] A laundry workers' union in St. Louis, Missouri, cautioned the patrons of Chinese washhouses that they ran "a great risk of contracting leprosy. . . . Chinese washhouses are already responsible for many cases of this loathsome disease among Americans."[15] Even the former head of the Louisiana Board of Health, Dr. Joseph Jones, warned that the "filthy" and "unprincipled, vicious and leprous hordes of Asia" could spread leprosy from the Far East to California and even Louisiana. Jones insisted that Chinese laundrymen were "in the early stages of the disease; and their practice of taking water in their mouths and spitting it out on the clothes they iron, is more than ever disgusting when considered in connection with the possible transmission of disease by this means."[16]

No matter that very few Chinese immigrants lived in New Orleans or that most of those diagnosed with the disease were natives, like Clara Mertz. People were worried. Hawaii was already grappling with a surge in leprosy cases and Americans feared they might be next. The highly publicized death in 1889 of Father Damien, a Catholic priest who contracted the disease while working with patients in a colony on the Hawaiian island of Molokai, fueled the mistaken belief that leprosy was highly contagious.[17] Reports that a Norwegian doctor had recently discovered a germ he believed caused the disease only bolstered that view.

Still, doctors at the time were divided, with many insisting that leprosy was hardly contagious and not nearly as dangerous as more common diseases, such as tuberculosis and smallpox. For decades, Louisianans had viewed leprosy as a serious illness, but one that could be treated at home or in a local hospital. Patients often lived in communities for years without anyone around them getting the disease. But the words of those who disagreed that leprosy was a significant threat fell on deaf ears. The *Picayune* even complained that the disagreement among medical experts was preventing a suitable response. "When doctors disagree so radically on matters of such great public importance, the only remedy is to appeal to common sense and reason, and enact proper protection for the people's health." The paper had an easy solution. The state should simply "declare" that leprosy was contagious, so victims could be quarantined.[18]

The *Picayune* continued to press its case, issuing one alarm after another, some of them false. "Laundresses and seamstresses who handle the clothing of lepers are most commonly infected by the scratch of a pin or the prick of a needle," the newspaper warned.[19] Kendall reported that the pesthouse cook, who had leprosy, was seen touching meat on a butcher's cart before deciding what to buy. The butcher then went around the corner and sold neighborhood families "the very meat the leper cook has handled and fumbled over."[20] That was the final straw. Something had to be done.

Isadore Dyer, a young New Orleans dermatologist, saw all the confusion and controversy as an opportunity to act. He was among those in the medical community who felt that leprosy, while only mildly contagious, was a growing threat. Dyer was twenty-eight but looked much older, with his receding hairline and plump jowls. He was also serious and intense, and well on his way to becoming one of the most influential voices in the city. Dyer had received his medical degree from Tulane and recently returned to the city after interning at the New York Skin and Cancer Hospital and studying in London and Paris.[21] He would soon be named dean of Tulane's medical school.[22]

But Dyer was more than a doctor. He was also a poet, philosopher, and public servant. Dyer had been raised in a Jewish family where accomplishment and service were highly prized. His aunt was one of the wealthiest philanthropists in the country, and had nursed Civil War soldiers and victims of yellow fever.[23] Dyer hoped to make his mark on the world as well. He wrote inspirational sayings in his diary, such as "Time is measured by the shadows of accomplisht tasks" and "No healthy man is a pessimist." He also composed a daily reminder, called "Each Day," that opened with the line: "Claim no other creed than faith expressed in service to those who are in need, forgetting self and building everyday a surer foundation for the everlasting brotherhood of man."[24] Dyer wanted to help some of society's neediest, the victims of leprosy. He thought the best way to do that was to segregate patients in a healthy environment, while conducting research for a cure.

Not surprisingly, he was appalled by the conditions at Dr. Beard's pesthouse. Seizing on the outrage that followed Kendall's reports, Dyer and another member of the Orleans Parish Medical Society called on the state legislature to toughen a law that already required the segregation of leprosy patients but was never enforced. The two men asked the legislature to establish a "place of detention . . . based upon the highest humanitarian plane" where patients would find an "asylum of refuge, rather than one of horror and reproach."[25] Dyer envisioned a hospital where leprosy patients would get humane, modern care, but also where doctors like himself could study the disease. Under growing pressure to act, the legislature in 1894 created the Louisiana Leper Home Board of Control, and Dyer was put in charge.[26]

The young dermatologist's first challenge was to find a location for the new home. Dyer wanted to put it in New Orleans, where patients would have access to the most up-to-date medical care. The Leper Home Board quickly identified several possible sites in the Crescent City, but when word got out, the neighbors protested. Over the course of the campaign to create a leprosy hospital, the public had become increasingly convinced that the disease posed a serious threat. Residents complained that their health would be at risk if the new hospital were located too close to their homes. They were especially disturbed that the board wanted to bring patients in from around the state. Dyer had estimated that there were about three hundred leprosy cases in Louisiana, with about a hundred in New Orleans. He argued that it made sense to put the home near where most of the patients already lived. New Orleanians thought otherwise.[27]

On the night of November 16, 1894, protesters filled City Hall, an imposing three-story marble building on Lafayette Square next to the French Quarter. They entered through a massive doorway, beneath a pediment on which three carved figures depicted Liberty, Commerce, and Justice. Five years earlier thousands of mourners had gathered at the same site to view the former president of the Confederacy, Jefferson Davis, whose body lay in state in the council chamber. Now residents gathered for a different, albeit less significant, cause, although some truly believed their lives were at stake. The protesters wanted the city council's public health committee to reject the Leper Home Board's recommendation that the new home be built inside city limits on Gentilly Road. Judge Walker, a spokesman for the neighborhood group, argued that the entire community could be infected with leprosy and that property values would certainly decline. He accused the Leper Home Board members—Dyer in particular—of wanting to locate the hospital nearby for their own convenience.

When Walker was done, Dyer rose to defend the board's selection. The doctor had a commanding presence, with his gold pocket-watch chain almost certainly draped across the vest of his three-piece suit. His posture announced that here was a man with serious medical credentials who should not be questioned. Dyer told the council members that leprosy was not nearly as contagious as the protesters believed. He insisted the disease could be spread only by close contact with an open wound (although that would later prove to be false). Dyer said it was also curious that city residents were suddenly so horrified by the disease, when not so long ago people with leprosy routinely rode on streetcars and ate in restaurants, with little fuss. These patients were their friends and neighbors, who deserved to be treated humanely. Dyer had no reason to believe his arguments would fail. He pleaded with the council to act quickly and approve the site because, he said, the patients at Dr. Beard's pesthouse were "dying of neglect." Unmoved, the committee denied his request.[28]

Dyer was now desperate. Dr. Beard, in response to the public outcry over conditions at the pesthouse, had submitted his resignation and the fate of the patients was unclear. One of the other board members, Captain Allen Jumel, had a possible solution. He lived in Iberville Parish, about seventy miles west of the city, and knew of an abandoned sugar plantation along the Mississippi River. The plantation, called Indian Camp, was isolated and swampy—not an ideal place to care for the sick—but it was available to lease for just $750 a year. The board had little choice. It declared the 350-acre site desirable in every way "except from the point of accessibility" and signed a five-year lease. Dyer and the others believed the arrangement would be temporary until they could find a permanent site for the home. To be safe, the plantation's neighbors were told that the new tenant planned to turn the property into an ostrich farm.

On the evening of November 30, Clara Mertz and six other patients at the pesthouse were picked up by a wagon driver and taken with their meager belongings to a coal barge waiting at the end of Lafayette Street. It was the only means of transportation the Leper Home Board could secure to move the patients to their new home. A ticket agent for the Texas and Pacific Railway Company had rejected their request for help with a typical excuse: "You can probably realize that should we charter a car or coach and use it for any other purpose afterwards, it might be the means of spreading the disease."[29] The crew on the tugboat hired to tow the barge upriver was also nervous and insisted that the ailing passengers be kept as far away from them as possible.[30] With that agreed upon, the barge was loaded with supplies, including several months' worth of food and bedding for the patients.

Mertz was the first patient to be helped out of the wagon and onto the barge. "At present she is suffering from a complication of diseases and her general appearance denotes the fact that she will not live long enough to derive the full benefits of the new home," wrote a reporter who was there to chronicle the occasion. The other patients—a woman and five men—followed Mertz and were soon joined by Dyer and several newspapermen for the overnight trip. With a blast of its whistle, the tug set off, pulling the barge into the dark. One of the reporters wrote that the tarp-covered barge "reminded one of the older stories of floating funerals, sorry laden vessels gliding down the Nile to the cities of the dead."[31]

Shortly before dawn, the barge arrived at a landing near Indian Camp, where the air was still and the darkness felt ominous. The passengers saw no sign of life, only a low earthen levee that lined the river and a dirt path that presumably led to the plantation. "It was thought by some that the place was as desolate as a desert," wrote one of the reporters. But as Dyer and a member of the crew climbed out to look around, a familiar figure suddenly emerged from the dark. Board member Jumel, with his bushy white beard and thick brows, looked like a "lord of the land" as he rode up on his horse. "Darn it boys, I am glad you came," he shouted out.

Jumel's greeting was a welcome relief, but the accommodations were not. When the passengers finally made their way over the levee and onto the property, they saw that the thirty-room plantation house was uninhabitable. Its exterior was filthy and chipped, its shutters and windows broken and grimy. Six crumbling Corinthian columns on the second-floor balcony hinted at the mansion's more opulent past, when the plantation was an active sugar farm and the site of frequent, lavish parties.[32] The patients were taken past the plantation house to seven wooden cabins out back where the plantation's slaves had once lived. The structures were rotting and leaky, but in slightly better shape than the house and would have to do. Dyer planned to hire a resident physician to care for Mertz and her fellow patients, but until then they were on their own, just as they had been in New Orleans. Only now they were much farther away from public view and the possibility of medical help.

On the riverbank that morning, a ten-year-old boy named Louis Arthur Carville had been sitting on his pony waiting for the barge to arrive. He and a local man were eager to see the ostriches that everyone in town expected to arrive. When they instead saw several "drab looking" people getting off the barge, a couple of them carried on stretchers, the man turned to the boy and said, "Lordy, Lordy, little Boss, them's no ostriches—them's sick folks." Another community would soon be enraged.[33]

Chapter 2

God versus Germs

IT IS NO wonder that people were terrified of leprosy. Victims' faces could be deformed by ugly nodules that clustered below the skin's surface like an army of thick, angry worms. Foreheads could be squeezed into deep frowns, and lips and ears could appear to have bubbled up like boiling soup. Noses could collapse into sinkholes. Some victims went blind or lost feeling in their hands and feet, leading to serious burns and infections. Fingers and toes might stiffen and shrink, as though snapped off at the knuckles, leaving only tiny stubs behind. Other victims suffocated as their windpipes swelled with infection.

The disease invaded slowly and surreptitiously, revealing itself first with seemingly harmless blemishes or the gentle tingling of fingers and toes. Conditions would usually worsen with time, becoming increasingly brutal and disabling, although seldom fatal. The victim was more likely to face a long life of pain and discomfort than a quick, merciful death. Many patients showed no obvious symptoms, but it was the most repulsive signs of leprosy that shaped people's response. It certainly looked like the punishment of a vengeful God.

For centuries, humanity mythologized this disease like no other. The Bible tied leprosy to sin and instructed priests to punish the sinner, in words that would resonate for centuries. "His clothes shall be torn and his head bare," said Leviticus. "And he shall cover his mustache, and cry, 'Unclean, Unclean!' He shall be unclean. All the days he has the sore he shall be unclean. He is unclean, and he shall dwell alone; his dwelling shall be outside the camp."[1] It was seen as a moral affliction as much as a physical one, and not just for readers of the Bible. Leprosy, with its terrifying power to deform, was considered to be a sign of evil. Hindus thought it resulted from misdeeds in a previous life. The Chinese believed it was divine punishment for necrophilia or sex with a prostitute. Pacific Islanders feared that it resulted from contact with a menstruating woman.[2]

This was a disease unlike any other—frightful, confusing, and loaded with mystical baggage. No matter that the leprosy of the Bible bore little, if any, resemblance to the disease that afflicted Clara Mertz and the others towed up the Mississippi River under the cover of night. Scholars now believe that biblical "leprosy" refers to a range of skin ailments, such as vitiligo, psoriasis, and ringworm. Leprous sores in the Bible are "white as snow," while blemishes in modern-day leprosy, or Hansen's disease, are more likely to be pink or red. In Leviticus, leprosy spreads to clothing and walls, leaving reddish and green stains, which is never the case with Hansen's disease. The Bible says a priest could determine whether someone was leprous by checking the afflicted person's skin after seven days of isolation. Hansen's disease symptoms take years to emerge. The Bible also never mentions the most common symptoms of the disease—blindness, numbness, and crippled hands.

It seems there was an unfortunate mistake in translation.

When the Greeks translated the Hebrew word *Tzaraath*, used in the Bible for "defiling skin diseases," they used *lepra*, meaning "scaly conditions." The Greeks had another name—"elephantiasis graecorum"—for the illness that would later become known as leprosy or Hansen's disease.[3] Over the centuries, one word morphed into another, and the leprosy of the Bible, and the stigma it entailed, became synonymous with the modern disease. As one Carville patient lamented, *leprosy* was once the word to describe many illnesses; all but one of them escaped.[4]

The victims of the disease paid a devastating price. Leprosy was feared not only for the physical impairment it caused but because victims were suspected of infecting others with their supposedly immoral ways. Medieval physicians thought those who had leprosy suffered from psychological deficiencies. They were schemers and deceivers, prone to uncontrolled sexual desire, who deserved to be isolated and scorned for the sake of the public's physical and moral well-being.[5]

As a result, those declared "lepers" in medieval times were often condemned to a spiritual death. A separation ritual, or Mass, made that abundantly clear. The victims would have their heads covered in veils and were required to kneel before an altar—or sometimes in an open grave, where a priest would throw dirt on their heads— so they could be banished from everyday life. They were no longer allowed to enter a church, marketplace, or tavern. They could not touch a child or use dishes and utensils other than their own. They were required to cover their bodies in robes and gloves, and carry a bell or clapper to warn others of their approach. Some victims were escorted to huts outside of town where they were isolated for the rest of their lives. There was no cure and therefore little hope for forgiveness and salvation. The only solace might be a priest's assurance that those afflicted with the disease would be rewarded in heaven for bearing such terrible suffering on earth.[6]

Still, the fate of those suspected of having leprosy often depended on who they were, who they knew, and where they lived. The rich and well connected usually fared better than the poor. It also depended on the politics of the day and the whims of the elite. Edward I of England had suspected lepers taken to a cemetery and buried alive. Philip V of France burned them at the stake.[7] But when leprous soldiers returned from the Crusades they were seen as the victims of foreign infection, not as sinners themselves.[8]

The diagnosis was also confusing and arbitrary. It was difficult to distinguish the disease from other ailments, such as syphilis, scabies, or psoriasis. Even in modern times, doctors can be confused, but in the Middle Ages, identifying leprosy was especially troublesome and prone to error. A priest or public official, not a doctor, usually decided. This person could easily be wrong, or vindictive, using the diagnosis to punish someone he disliked.[9]

The world of the "leper" has always been one of contradiction and inconsistency. Victims were simultaneously pitied and scorned, protected and shunned.[10] Many patients were treated humanely at some of the thousands of asylums that emerged outside city gates in medieval Europe. They received clothing, food, and medical care, often from the very same Church that had cast them out. These leprosaria became sanctuaries as well as prisons, harboring patients from the cruelty of others.[11] Centuries later, Carville would fill a similar role.

No one is sure why, but leprosy had all but disappeared from Europe by the 1500s. Better living conditions and diet, and the emergence of more devastating diseases, likely played a role. But the mythology and stigma lived on, simmering beneath the surface for centuries, waiting to reemerge when the time was ripe. That turned out to be the late 1800s, when massive migration and global exploration were rapidly reshaping and unsettling the world. People were mixing in unprecedented ways, creating new opportunities to spread illness and fear.[12]

A new book, published in 1880, reignited the old superstitions. *Ben-Hur: A Tale of the Christ* affirmed the belief that those afflicted with leprosy were cursed by God and that only the faithful could be cured. "We are lepers, and have no homes; we belong to the dead," Ben-Hur's sister Tirzah cries in despair as she and her mother are banished from Jerusalem. Author Lew Wallace describes their appearance in agonizing detail. "The eyelids, the lips, the nostrils, the flesh of the cheeks, were either gone or reduced to fetid rawness. . . . The nails had been eaten away; the joints of the fingers, if not bare to the bone, were swollen knots crusted with red secretion."[13] The symptoms disappear when the women are miraculously cured by Jesus Christ. *Ben-Hur* was a best seller for decades, and for a time was second only to the Bible in popularity.

Western missionaries helped to perpetuate the myths. As they traveled the world to spread Christian beliefs, they turned their attention and fundraising campaigns to the victims of leprosy, seen as some of the most destitute people on earth. Sympathetic Christians donated money to help the "unfortunates" and, they hoped, to save their souls. It was a well-intentioned gesture that again linked leprosy to sin. Belief in God was considered a surefire path to salvation and relief. Wellesley Bailey, who founded the British Mission to Lepers in 1874, was convinced—after visiting patients in India —that their "first and greatest need was the Gospel."[14]

———

A young doctor in Norway at the time strongly disagreed. Gerhard Henrik Armauer Hansen, an avowed atheist, thought that what the victims of leprosy needed most was a cure. He was part of a new generation of physicians who believed that diseases were caused by tiny organisms called "germs," and that if those pathogens could be identified, a disease might be controlled and even cured. Like Isadore Dyer in Louisiana, Hansen was extremely ambitious. He longed to be on the cutting edge of modern medicine and the emerging field of microbiology. He was eager to prove both his theories and himself.

Hansen was one of fifteen children who grew up in a middle-class family in Bergen, a busy port on the west coast of Norway, a country with a surprisingly high rate of leprosy. No one knew why that was the case, but the young Hansen was intrigued. He received his medical degree in 1866 and went north to the remote Lofoten Islands to care for cod fishermen. But he soon returned home for a chance to work with one of the world's leading experts on leprosy. Dr. Daniel Cornelius Danielssen headed research at two of the three hospitals in Bergen devoted to patients with the disease. Danielssen was among those trying to determine why almost three thousand Norwegians had leprosy, more than in any other European country. The disease had been present since Viking times but it appeared to be spreading, especially among fishermen and peasants. Norway was one of the poorest countries in Europe and Danielssen believed that unsanitary and stressful living conditions contributed to what was primarily a hereditary disease.[15]

Hansen was not convinced. The young doctor noticed that in areas where leprosy patients had been segregated in hospitals—primarily to keep them from marrying and having children who might perpetuate the disease—the number of cases had declined. To him, this was a sign that leprosy was more likely contagious than hereditary.

This put Hansen at odds with his new boss, who had written what was considered to be the definitive book on the disease, called *On Leprosy*. Danielssen and coauthor C. W. Boeck were the first in the world to describe leprosy in medical terms and to distinguish it from other illnesses. They also identified the two forms of leprosy that would be recognized for decades to come—tuberculoid and lepromatous.[16] The first form was milder and less contagious than the second. It produced skin lesions and numbness but was not as physically invasive as lepromatous leprosy, which caused far greater damage to nerves, skin, and organs such as the eyes. Danielssen was convinced that leprosy was not contagious because he had tried repeatedly to inoculate himself and his assistants with leprous tissue. Try as he might, he could not give himself the disease. As far as he was concerned, the case was closed, but he encouraged Hansen—who had just married Danielssen's daughter—to pursue his theory.[17]

Hansen believed that extensive data collected by Norwegian health authorities would back him up. The country had set up a first-of-its-kind registry, which tracked leprosy patients by age, gender, place of birth, and whether any close relatives had the disease. But he also needed physical proof.

The young doctor began to study tissue samples from some of the two hundred patients at the hospital where he worked. Hansen was a researcher at heart, far more comfortable in the lab than at the bedsides of those he was trying to help, although he said he was motivated by seeing "so much misery concentrated in one place."[18] With his eyes glued to a microscope, his long, scraggly beard dangling down, the thirty-two-year-old doctor spent hours scouring slide after slide for clues. Finally, on February 28, 1873, he spotted something in one of the samples that would eventually reshape medical thinking. He saw tiny rod-shaped bodies that he believed to be the bacteria responsible for causing leprosy.[19] But Hansen was extremely cautious about trumpeting his findings. "Though unable to discover any difference between these bodies and true bacteria, I will not venture to declare them to be actually identical," he reported.[20]

Hansen was hesitant because he had yet to meet a crucial scientific test at the time for proving that a germ caused a particular illness. That test required that he be able to cultivate the bacteria in a lab and then use them to transmit the disease to another person or an animal. Hansen tried desperately to do so for several years after his initial discovery, without success, using rabbits as subjects. He became increasingly frustrated, and then angry when a German researcher who had visited and reviewed Hansen's work returned home and published a paper in which he seemed to take credit for Hansen's discovery.[21]

Desperate, the Norwegian doctor made a last-ditch attempt to prove his theory. On November 3, 1879, Hansen asked a woman who had been a patient at the hospital for seventeen years to come into his examining room. Kari Nielsdatter Spidsøen suffered from the milder, tuberculoid form of the disease, and Hansen speculated that if he could infect the thirty-three-year-old woman with tissue from a patient who suffered from the more severe lepromatous form, he would be able to show that the disease was contagious. He decided not to ask the young woman for her permission to perform the experiment.

Spidsøen was nervous as soon as she entered Hansen's office and saw two other doctors waiting there with him. She then noticed that Hansen held a cataract knife, a long, thin tool that looked like a needle. The woman began to cry and became frantic when he tried to insert the knife into her left eye. She held up one arm to shield her face and pushed Hansen away with the other. One of the other doctors tried to subdue Spidsøen and eventually got her into a chair. He held her there as Hansen used the knife to insert the leprous tissue under the conjunctiva, or outer membrane, of her eye. Hansen assured Spidsøen that she would be fine, but the weeping woman pleaded with him not to cut into her other eye, and he agreed.

Spidsøen complained for weeks that she was in pain and had

trouble seeing. Other patients were upset by the incident and a minister at the hospital finally reported it to authorities. Human experimentation was not uncommon at the time, but conducting it without a subject's consent was. Hansen was taken to court.

The trial did not go smoothly—for Spidsøen. One of the doctors told the judge that the patient had only imagined her pain and the procedure was harmless. He dismissed the woman as a "nervous and hysterical subject." When Hansen took the witness stand, he argued that since Spidsøen already had leprosy, he was not infecting her with a new disease, merely a different form of something she already had. He said he was confident that he could remove any leprous growth on her eye that might result, although none ever did. Hansen admitted to the judge that he probably should have told Spidsøen what he planned to do and asked for her permission, but he had assumed she would object. He said that he proceeded anyway because the goal of finding the cause of leprosy was of such "great scientific and national importance."[22]

The court was sympathetic. Members of the medical establishment believed that Hansen's actions were justified and that the welfare of individual leprosy patients—who tended to be poor—could be sacrificed for the greater good. The head of the Norwegian Health Directorate noted that "the experiment had been carried out to contribute to a question with the most important consequences for science, the nation and the patients." While "the patient had not given her distinct permission for the operation, she had on the other hand not distinctly opposed it."[23]

Hansen was punished, but the punishment was light. He lost his position as resident physician at the hospital but was allowed to remain Norway's chief medical officer for leprosy. He could pursue his research, although not on human subjects. Kari Spidsøen asked to be transferred to a new hospital after the incident. She was moved two years later, and died shortly thereafter.

Even though he was unable to prove his theory in the lab, Hansen remained convinced that leprosy was contagious and that segregating patients was the best way to contain the disease.[24] He also believed that "healthy people must have the same humane treatment as the sick" and that authorities had the right and duty to isolate the sick if they posed a threat to the community.[25] His ideas gained traction within the medical community and in 1885 Norway passed the Act on the Seclusion of Lepers, which required patients to be confined either at home or in a hospital. Hansen, the man of science, ended up promoting a strategy that was not all that different from the one favored centuries earlier by the men of God.

It would be decades before health experts realized that this strategy was seriously flawed. Leprosy's long incubation period meant that it could be years before those infected with the disease were diagnosed. By that time, the damage was done. If the infected individual had been close to someone prone to leprosy—such as a sibling—the germ had likely already spread. Instead, the threat of being exiled, possibly for life, discouraged those who suspected they might have leprosy from seeking help.

But Norway's approach attracted international attention, largely because the new segregation policy coincided with a rapid decline of the disease. Norway had registered 1,040 new cases of leprosy in 1861. By 1896, that number was down to 89. Some experts suspected that better living conditions were the real reason for the drop, but doctors around the world took note.[26] Isadore Dyer was one of them. He was excited by Hansen's work and saw Norway as the model for what he hoped to achieve in Louisiana. He wanted a first-rate hospital where patients would be isolated but could still receive humane care and benefit from the latest medical research. He quickly discovered how easily such well-intentioned plans could be derailed.

Chapter 3

Rescue Mission

ISADORE DYER WAS frustrated. The mosquito-infested property along the Mississippi River was not at all what he had imagined for his new leprosy hospital. It was certainly nothing like what the *Daily Picayune* described shortly after the first residents arrived. "There is not one among the seven patients who left the Hagan Avenue pesthole who regrets going to the new place where every comfort is at hand and a kind voice soothes them when suffering impels them to complain." The newspaper said the patients now lived in big, "comfortable cabins, surrounded by massive oaks" behind a grand mansion with pillars across the front "crowned by Corinthian capitals of great beauty."[1]

On the surface, there was some truth to that. The old plantation was indeed hauntingly beautiful, green and lush. The live oak trees, with their twisted limbs dripping in Spanish moss, provided refreshing tents of shade. The air was filled with the calls of thousands of birds hidden in their branches—blue jays, mockingbirds, woodpeckers, and hawks. But there were also alligators and snakes hiding in the mud and weeds. In summer, mosquitoes would attack with astounding ferocity. Everything that made the area perfect for growing sugarcane—the heat, humidity, and relentless rain— made it unsuitable for living. The old mansion, once so elegant that visitors stayed for weeks at a time to enjoy its splendor, was overrun by bats and vermin. The slave cabins, where the patients were housed, offered little protection from the wind and the rain. "Everything around spoke of decay and ruin," a visitor wrote.[2]

It seemed fitting that the exiled patients had been placed in cabins where others had been shunned and dehumanized before them. Only a few decades earlier, dozens of slaves were forced to toil under the brutal conditions of a Louisiana sugar farm, planting, harvesting, and grinding the stalks that would eventually become the granulated sugar and molasses stacked on the New Orleans docks. The slaves were literally worked to death, often within a few years of arriving at the farm. The scent of death and failure was all around. The plantation owner, Robert Camp, was a bachelor who gave extravagant parties, but he was not a good businessman. He was constantly in debt, and creditors finally seized the property after the Civil War, which led to its abandonment and decline.

The patients' lives were not nearly as brutal as those of the slaves, but they also found themselves surrounded by hardship and hate. The residents of Iberville Parish were furious when they learned they had been fooled and their new neighbors were not ostriches but society's outcasts. Local merchants refused to deliver food and supplies to the home. Black laborers hired to work there were warned that they would be shot if they left the property.[3] Nothing was going as planned and Dyer's vision of a modern sanitarium appeared doomed from the start. "At every hand obstacles were thrown in the way of the Board's efforts to fulfill the high duty imposed upon them," he later complained.[4]

So it was not a complete surprise when a group of angry men showed up unannounced at the board's New Orleans office soon after the first patients arrived. Eight members of Iberville Parish's governing body, called the "police jury," had come to confront the board. They wanted the "lepers" gone. The men complained that the patients' presence threatened the health of parish residents and would depress their property values—the same arguments the board had heard only a few weeks earlier from residents of New Orleans.[5] But the board had little choice and refused to budge. They challenged the Iberville men to come up with a better site for the home and asked if they'd be willing to reimburse the state for the rent it had already paid on Indian Camp. If not, the home was there to stay. Dyer and the other board members also warned the police jury that if there was even a hint of violence, state troopers would be sent in to defend the home. The men from Iberville left, vowing to take their fight to court.

The board was in a bind, one of its own making. Dyer and the others had insisted that leprosy was such a serious threat to public health that the patients needed to be segregated. But at the same time, the board needed to convince people that the disease was not contagious enough for those living nearby to worry about infection. The public was understandably confused. The next day, the *Daily Picayune* weighed in, criticizing Iberville residents for being so unreasonable. The newspaper insisted that the presence of leprosy patients in New Orleans over the years had never discouraged visitors or depressed property values. The paper conveniently ignored the fact that the Leper Home's current remote location was due in part to the newspaper's overwrought coverage. The *Picayune* asked Iberville residents to have "pity for the unfortunates" because they had to live somewhere "since there is no law by which they can be exterminated."[6]

The Iberville police jury sent Dyer an offer several days later.

The parish would pay the state $750 to move the home. The board rejected the plan because it had nowhere else to go.[7]

Back at the plantation, things were not going well at all. A doctor, L. A. Wailes, had been hired to care for the patients and manage the property, but he was immediately overwhelmed. Wailes complained a few weeks into the job that there was no clean water for bathing and treating the patients' wounds and that the residents' health was already deteriorating. He said some of them showed signs of malaria. Others, whose hands were numbed by the disease, had burned themselves on the fires they kept in their cabins for cooking and heat. "At this time, the patients do not present a very cheerful or encouraging appearance," he informed the board.[8] The only good news was that the old slave cabins had been whitewashed and broken planks of wood had been replaced. A school in New Orleans had donated books and food for the patients and shelves had been installed in one of the cabins for a "leper's library." The board also sent the patients musical instruments—a banjo, an accordion, and a concertina—so they could keep themselves entertained.

But things were moving far too slowly for Dyer. His plan to control the spread of leprosy depended on patients wanting to come to the home voluntarily so they could avoid infecting anyone else. If the home was not attractive, patients would refuse to go there. They would have to be forcibly confined, something he wanted to avoid. Doctors and sheriffs around the state had already shown little interest in enforcing the new state law, which technically required them to send anyone with leprosy to the home. Only in New Orleans did then-mayor John Fitzpatrick order the police to arrest any "lepers" they found roaming the streets for eventual exile to Indian Camp. But the officers balked at the order, worried that they would infect other prisoners or, worse, themselves.[9] Many doctors in the state also refused or failed to report suspected cases of the disease to the authorities. After all, these patients were their friends and neighbors, even relatives, who had lived in their communities for decades. It was one of the many contradictions the Leper Home Board had to contend with. Sometimes people feared leprosy, but sometimes they didn't.

Dyer decided to get more aggressive.[10] On January 25, 1895, less than two months after the home opened, he issued a proclamation that was printed in newspapers around the state. He warned of "the dangers of contagion, to which all are exposed by the increasing number of lepers in this state" and appealed for all citizens to cooperate with the new quarantine law. He presented the Leper Home in the best light, sounding like a desperate salesman trying to unload some property. The home on the Mississippi River was "accessible by boat and by railroad" and provided "the liberty and comforts which the imprisoned leper in his own desolate family life cannot enjoy." Dyer promised that "modern hospital methods are used, and the conveniences in the way of furniture and household materials [are] sufficient." He also reminded residents that it was a misdemeanor to harbor someone with leprosy and warned that if people did not come willingly, parish sheriffs would be called upon to enforce the law. "We are anxious to spare the individual leper the embarrassment and mortification with which the publicity of the legal procedure of committal is attended," he proclaimed. "We shall be glad, therefore, to receive all lepers at any time upon demand for admission, irrespective of race or color, age or sex."[11]

His proclamation had almost no impact. Dyer and other physicians on the board were able to cajole a few of their own leprosy patients to go to Indian Camp. But by May, there were only seventeen residents at the home.[12] If anything, the new law had forced some who suffered from the disease to flee into the state's remote swamplands to avoid being caught. They would now get no care at all, the opposite of what Dyer had intended.

Wailes's appeals to the board became increasingly desperate. Iberville Parish had quietly dropped its plans to challenge the board in court, but local merchants still refused to deliver supplies. "I am entirely out of flour, milk, and bacon," Wailes wrote in May. In June, he fired the home's cook and warned the board that he might have to fire two other employees for "drunkenness and disorderly conduct." He complained that patients were suffering from malaria, dysentery, and diarrhea, and that floodwaters threatened the home. Wailes signed one of his letters, "Yours in such tribulation!" and underlined each word for emphasis. When the first patient died at the end of June—a sixty-five-year-old man identified only as "J.D."—the doctor wrote that he was unable to find a priest willing to come to the home to bury him. By August, they were "entirely out of coffee & butter" and Wailes reported that a male nurse he had hired refused to touch the patients, making the nurse completely worthless. "I am worn out—literally & both mentally & physically & and must have help immediately," the doctor pleaded.[13]

Dyer realized something had to be done. Wailes was clearly in over his head and unable to oversee the care of the patients on his own. Dyer decided to seek help from the one organization he believed would be unable to refuse his request—the Catholic sisters who served as nurses at Charity Hospital in New Orleans. The Daughters of Charity were widely respected for their compassionate care of the sick and the poor, and had experience treating leprosy patients at the hospital. But the sisters were not eager to go to such a remote, ill-equipped place. Their superior in Emmitsburg, Maryland, Mother Mariana Flynn, told the board the sisters would accept the assignment only under certain conditions—that they be provided "proper" accommodations, a chaplain to conduct religious services, and a modest stipend for clothing and travel.[14]

The board assured her it would meet the demands, but the sisters were unwilling to take such a promise on faith. In February of 1896, Sister Agnes Slavin of Charity Hospital went to Indian Camp to check out the conditions for herself. Her difficult journey was not a promising sign. She had to take one train from New Orleans to Donaldson, about three-quarters of the way there, then another train to the tiny town of White Castle, across the river from Indian Camp. From there, she had to climb the levee to catch a small skiff to the opposite bank. It was so muddy that Sister Agnes borrowed the captain's rubber boots to get to the road, where she found a driver with a cart and an old horse to take her the last mile to the plantation gate.

What Sister Agnes found at the Leper Home was worse than she had expected. She reported back to Mother Mariana that the plantation mansion might have been "a palace in its time but is in such a ruinous state you could form no idea how it is." She said a small building where the sisters were intended to live was more like a chicken house, propped up on six-foot-high stilts above the swampy ground. "On the whole, I could not imagine anything so uncomfortable—there is only a single floor and when you are under the house you can see through the crevices," she wrote. "I would not think of letting the Sisters live in this house—they would lose their health and unless proper arrangements were made with sufficient room for baths, closets and sleeping room, let them wait," she wrote.[15]

The sisters would also have to walk through muddy fields to reach the patients, who were now confined to a twenty-two-acre area surrounded by an eight-foot-high fence. Sister Agnes said it would be especially difficult to get to them at night on the pitch-dark property. Two cabins were used for women patients and two for men, with about six to eight patients in each. Sister Agnes said the rooms were generally clean and the patients were comfortable, but they had no tubs to bathe in. When she asked one bedridden man if he'd seen a priest, he told her, "Oh, no, Sister, they won't come here." One cabin used as a kitchen was intended to be turned into a chapel, which Sister Agnes said "would not do in any way." She also reported that she was shocked to learn that male and female patients were allowed to socialize "even at night." The Daughters of Charity would not agree to come without considerable changes.

But the board had nowhere else to turn for help. Dyer appealed to a priest who oversaw the Daughters of Charity, and Sister Agnes was overruled. On March 25, 1896, the Leper Home Board of Control signed a contract with the Daughters of Charity to manage the home and care for the patients. Each sister would receive one hundred dollars a year for clothing and other expenses, but otherwise they would work for free. The board members hoped that now Louisianans with leprosy would be much more willing to go to the home, knowing they'd be under the sisters' good care.

A few weeks later, as the sun set over the Mississippi River, four Daughters of Charity walked up the plank of the *Paul Tulane*, a steamboat waiting to take them from New Orleans to Indian Camp. The women were hard to miss. Like all Daughters of Charity, they wore stiff white headpieces, called cornettes, which swooped into the air like the wings of a swan. Matching starched white collars covered their chests like shields. Beneath, they wore blue woolen robes that gathered in thick folds at their waists and dusted the ground as they walked. The women were led by fifty-five-year-old Sister Beatrice Hart, who had arrived from Lowell, Massachusetts, where she ran a hospital for twenty-two years. She was joined by three other women, all in their thirties—Sisters Annie Costello, Cyril Coupe, and Mary Thomas Stockum. All four had volunteered for the assignment, considered to be extremely hazardous even by those accustomed to working with the sick and the poor.[16]

Their send-off could hardly have been more different from the one two years earlier when the patients were secretly towed away in the dark. A large crowd had gathered on the dock to see the sisters depart, "bound for the leper land!" as the newspapers would later report. Men waved their hats in the air as the women stood on deck waving their white handkerchiefs in return. "It was something of the tribute that a hero receives when he goes forth with deathless courage to battle to the end and wrest victory in a cause that is all but lost," wrote the *Daily Picayune*.[17] Spectators on shore believed the sisters were headed to their doom.

―――――――

The women arrived at Indian Camp the following afternoon, and were greeted at the dock by Dr. Wailes and patients, who Sister Beatrice said "almost wept for joy" as the sisters approached. "They told us that you were coming, but we would not believe it," one patient said in a trembling voice. "Have you really, really come to stay with us?" asked another. Sister Beatrice reassured them that the sisters were there to stay. "And, dear friends, we do not intend to ever have the word 'leper' mentioned in our home again," she promised. "We are going to call you our friends—our patients." She was wrong about the word *leper*, which would be used repeatedly by her and others at the home for decades to come. But the residents had no way of knowing that. They were overjoyed that help had finally arrived.[18]

The sisters got down to business right away, going from cabin to cabin to assess conditions and to meet those too ill to come outside to greet them. There were now about thirty patients in all, ranging in age from ten to sixty. It was a sobering sight, even for those who were used to dealing with misery. In one cabin, they found four young women, all siblings. One of them said her bed sheets had been changed only twice in six months.[19]

There was much to do, but one thing took precedence. The Daughters of Charity were there to care for not only the patients' bodies but also their souls. The women brushed away dust and spider webs in an empty room and set up a makeshift chapel with liturgical supplies they had brought with them on the boat. That Sunday, Catholic Mass was held at the home for the first time. Sixteen patients attended the service, conducted by a priest who had been recruited to serve as the home's chaplain. "When he bade them lift up your hearts, sobs could be heard throughout the Chapel and we could not refrain from mingling our tears with theirs," Sister Beatrice recalled.[20] After Mass, the sisters organized a party for the patients with lemonade and cake.

The Daughters of Charity had their work cut out for them. Sister Agnes was right. The mansion was in complete disrepair. "The walls oozed moisture, the roof admitted torrents of rain, broken floors furnished shelter to rats, while unused attic and rooms were veritable havens for bats and snakes," a sister wrote. When one of the Daughters of Charity went to explore the house and opened a closet, she was startled to find a knot of snakes nested inside. Another sister tumbled from a second-story room when the floor beneath her collapsed. She saved herself by grabbing on to a piece of timber protruding from the wall. The women kept axes by their beds to kill water moccasins that sometimes climbed their bedposts at night.[21]

To make matters worse, Dr. Wailes quit within days of the sisters' arrival. The board hired a replacement, but he seldom came. The sisters now had to see to the patients' medical needs as well as make their meals, do laundry, and manage the home. It was far more than they had bargained for. A month after their arrival, a man hired to work at the home got drunk and used an ax to try to kill a young boy who also worked on the grounds.[22] "It was like an uncivilized wilderness," said one of the sisters.[23]

Still, the women did what they could. They set up a common dining room so patients no longer had to eat in their cabins. Sister Beatrice began soliciting donations from anyone willing to help the "unfortunates." A doctor from Charity Hospital shipped an organ to the home and a woman from White Castle, across the river, sent six dozen pillow cases and an assortment of delicacies, including canned pears, mustard, sardines, and pickles.[24] "I'm sort of a high minded beggar," Sister Beatrice wrote. "When they ask me what I want, I tell them the best, for I do not believe the patients should have anything less."[25] She encouraged the patients to keep busy, growing flowers, vegetables, and fruits and helping with domestic chores "to divert their minds from melancholy brooding over their unhappy condition." Besides music, croquet became a favorite pastime.[26] Sister Beatrice also promised to give the patients proper "Christian" burials, noting that previously they "were thrown like dogs into the grave the same day they died." She said the patients told her that the change had "taken away all the sting of dying here."[27]

A reporter who visited not long after the sisters' arrival wrote of a miraculous change. He said the cabins were "scrupulously neat and clean," with flowers on the mantels and snowy white coverlets on the beds. Every room was equipped with a pile of books and a rocking chair. Wooden walkways now connected the sisters' quarters and the patients' cabins, making it much easier to get from one to the other. "Oh, yes! ye lepers, wherever you are hiding to-day, there is hope and tenderness and gentle care awaiting you in the retreat which a kind government has provided in the settlement at White Castle. Do not fear to go there," the reporter wrote.[28]

With things looking up, Dyer proposed that the state purchase the plantation and make it the hospital's permanent home. While he still preferred a site closer to New Orleans, he was resigned to the fact that such a move was unlikely. At least if the state owned Indian Camp, he reasoned, lawmakers would be more inclined to

provide money to fix up the home. But representatives from Iberville Parish vehemently objected to keeping the Leper Home at
Indian Camp and the legislature rejected the plan. For Dyer, it was
a disheartening sign that the state had abandoned the patients. In
June of 1896, he and two other board members resigned in protest.[29] The resignations made national news, because Dyer's work
had started to attract attention from outside the state. The *New
York Sun* complained that Dyer would now be unable to pursue his
goal of testing possible treatments that he hoped would "secure, in
time, some remedy that would get rid of leprosy."[30]

After a few months on the job, Sister Beatrice was also getting restless. Even though conditions had started to improve, she
complained to Mother Mariana that not one member of the Leper
Home Board had come to see how things were going. So far from
the city, the home was too easy to ignore. When board members
finally visited in August, she pleaded with them to find someplace
less isolated and more conducive to providing decent medical
care.[31] She was secretly pleased to learn that the men had a difficult time getting home, which only reinforced her point about
the Leper Home's highly unsuitable location. The board members
were forced to wait in an open field in the hot sun to flag down the
only train available to take them back to New Orleans.[32]

There wasn't much the sisters could do to treat the patients,
other than to try to keep them clean and comfortable. The most
common treatment for leprosy at the time was largely worthless—
a daily dose of an oil from the tropical chaulmoogra tree. Some
patients thought the foul-smelling medicine eased their symptoms,
but most said it made them feel nauseated. The patients were also
sick with sorrow, abandoned as they were by relatives and friends.
"We received during the past week a little girl, an entire orphan,
and she seems so lonely and dispirited that my heart aches for the
child," wrote Sister Beatrice.[33] Like Wailes, Sister Beatrice had

trouble getting help. She said dentists refused to come to the home for fear it would destroy their businesses if word got out. She complained that one doctor hired to care for the patients was "really insane" and the patients refused to see him.[34]

Dyer, who was no longer on the board, accused its members of inaction and doing nothing to try to cure the disease.[35] He was especially disturbed because he had hoped that Louisiana—which had more cases of leprosy than anywhere else in the country— would be at the forefront of global efforts to fight the disease. In 1897 Dyer attended the first International Leprosy Conference in Berlin, where medical experts from around the world agreed to a resolution declaring that "every leper is a danger to his surroundings" and calling for compulsory isolation. The author of the resolution was Norway's Dr. Hansen.[36] His discovery of the *Mycobacterium leprae* germ had given doctors hope that they might finally wrestle to the ground one of humankind's oldest diseases. But it looked less and less likely that Louisiana would play a role.

The members of the Leper Home Board, in fact, wanted to move the home but were having a difficult time finding a suitable site.[37] In the spring of 1901, they finally located what looked like the perfect spot, another abandoned plantation along the Mississippi River but much closer to New Orleans. The four-hundred-acre Elkhorn Plantation was in Jefferson Parish, right outside city limits and convenient to a rail line. Doctors from Tulane and Charity Hospital could easily get there to treat the patients. The board purchased the property, but did so in secret, unwilling to risk another uprising. The seller was told that the land was to be used for a truck farm and fruit orchard.

But word got out anyway and residents were predictably furious. They called the state's plan to put a "leper" home in their parish "an outrage no community should be called upon to endure." One man proposed that the patients be confined instead on an island off the Gulf Coast.[38] Board members tried to reassure residents that they would not be at risk of contagion. The *Picayune* argued that they were in more danger of contracting the disease from the hundreds of leprosy patients walking around the state untreated because they refused to go somewhere as remote as Indian Camp.[39]

The arguments fell on deaf ears. Rumors started to spread that a ferry was on its way to Indian Camp to pick up the patients and bring them to Elkhorn Plantation.[40] On May 22, 1901, the Leper Home Board of Control met with a dozen representatives of Jefferson and nearby St. Charles Parishes to calm things down, but the residents left the meeting unmoved. One man said the home would never be allowed inside the parish under any conditions. That night, the issue was resolved. Shortly after midnight, the sky over the deserted plantation lit up like a giant flare as the main house became engulfed in fire. Soon after, two small outhouses burst into flames, and no one came to put them out. By morning, there was nothing left but charred remains.[41]

The board had little choice but to stay at Indian Camp. By that summer, the sisters were sick and exhausted. Sister Beatrice was struck with malaria but continued to work despite being critically ill. She spent the night with a dying patient before she finally took to her bed in the mansion, where she had to be moved from one side of her room to the other "as the rain, driven by the wind, came in first from one direction and then from another."[42] The woman who had been so optimistic five years earlier when she arrived at Indian Camp was resigned to her fate and that of her fellow sisters and patients. Caring for those with leprosy did not seem to be a high priority for anyone. She had complained to the board in August that the latest doctor hired to treat the patients showed up only once or twice a month. "But what can you do," she wrote. "There is no one else to be had."[43] Five weeks later, Sister Beatrice was dead.

Chapter 4

Rebellion

THE SAME DAY that Sister Beatrice died in Louisiana the nation was shaken by another death. President William McKinley succumbed to his wounds on the morning of September 14, 1901, a week after being shot by an assassin at the Pan-American Exposition in Buffalo, New York. The fair was intended to be a celebration of American greatness and technological know-how, and more than a hundred thousand people showed up to hear the popular twenty-fifth president speak. The United States was basking in its victory in the Spanish-American War and there seemed to be no limit to what the country could achieve. The crowd at the fair was treated to a rousing concert by John Philip Sousa and an extravagant fireworks show. Fairgoers watched in awe as the words "Welcome President McKinley, Chief of Our Nation and Our Empire" splashed across the sky in glittering lights. The following day, the president returned to the fair and, as he shook hands with well-wishers at the Temple of Music, was shot by an anarchist. It looked like the president might recover, but eight days later he died from gangrene.

The new president—Vice President Theodore Roosevelt—was eager to expand the American empire even further. He was sworn in later that day, after being pulled from a family camping trip in the Adirondacks. The forty-two-year-old Roosevelt was the nation's youngest president so far and brought an energy and swagger to the office that would be felt around the world and eventually in a remote leprosarium in Louisiana. As the leader of a cavalry regiment called the Rough Riders, he had inspired thousands of young men to enlist three years earlier in the U.S. effort to oust Spain from Cuba and to end its colonial rule of the Philippines. Now he needed more troops to secure U.S. control of the Southeast Asian nation, where rebels continued to resist the Americans.

So it is no surprise that two days after McKinley's death, a cocky sixteen-year-old butcher walked into a recruiter's office in New Haven, Connecticut, and signed up to join the army. Morris Kolnitzky had many reasons to do so. He wanted to escape the grip of his overbearing, extremely religious Jewish father. He was also an ambitious young man, likely motivated by the new president's thirst for adventure and glory. Traveling halfway around the globe to fight the enemies of democracy seemed far more exciting than cutting up animal carcasses in New Haven.

Kolnitzky was so eager to enlist that he lied about his age. He was supposed to be at least eighteen years old to sign up, but he said he was twenty-one and a half so he would not need his parents' permission. Apparently, the recruiter never bothered to check. Kolnitzky was just the kind of soldier the army could use, a young man packed with power and determination. He was only five-foot-four but extremely strong for his size. He also looked much older than his age, with dark, piercing eyes and only a hint of baby fat left in his cheeks. The recruiter also didn't bother to check Kolnitzky's name. Whether by mistake or design, the young man was enlisted as "Kolnsky," the name that would appear on his gravestone thirty-seven years later. One thing on his enlistment papers was accurate. He was born in Odessa, Russia, from which his family had emigrated a decade earlier.

On January 23, 1902, Kolnitzky and hundreds of other fresh recruits in the 27th Infantry set off for the Philippines from New York Harbor on the transport ship *Buford*. The trip to Manila Bay took almost two months, and as soon as they arrived, the young men were sent several hundred miles south to the island of Mindanao. The area around Mindanao's massive Lake Lanao was one of the last, and most brutal, rebel holdouts. Two American soldiers had recently been murdered on the island—one of them hacked to death when he went out for a stroll—and U.S. authorities believed the Moro Muslims who lived near Lake Lanao were responsible. The 27th Infantry had been picked to join an expedition to retaliate.[1]

Like Kolnitzky, most of the soldiers had never seen battle before. They were already exhausted when they set out on a grueling trek through thick jungle terrain to find the intended target. Their commander, Colonel Frank Baldwin, had been ordered to avoid fighting the Moros if possible, because President Roosevelt wanted to declare soon that the insurrection was over and new hostilities could derail that plan. But Baldwin was headstrong and intent on punishing the Moros for the Americans' deaths. The expedition began with over a thousand men, but many of them were quickly overcome by extreme heat, fatigue, and illness, and had to turn back. The march became more difficult when Filipino Muslims, who had been hired by the army as porters, discovered that the American supplies included cans of pork. They immediately dropped their loads and fled. The six hundred remaining men slowly made their way along a narrow footpath, rutted with ditches and cluttered with fallen trees. It took them seventeen days to complete the thirty-two-mile trail to Lake Lanao. By the time they reached their destination, the village of Bayan, supplies were short and many of the men were weakened by dysentery.[2]

The Americans found the Moros in two forts sitting on separate hills overlooking the lake. The infantrymen quickly seized the smaller fort, driving the rebels to the second, larger one, where red battle flags flew high above the outer wall. Hundreds of Moros were positioned inside. This was where the real fight would be waged. As U.S. mountain guns hurled shells overhead, about three hundred infantrymen stormed up the hill. When they neared the top, dozens of sword-swinging rebels emerged from trenches that surrounded the fort. The infantrymen fought back desperately with rifles, bayonets, and anything else they could find. "It was shoot, cut, bite, throw rocks and yell," one soldier reported from the front. By the end, "the Moros in the trenches were all dead, but our loss was heavy."[3]

The Americans struggled on, making their way around booby-trapped ditches. They tried to scale the walls of the fort but were driven back by gunfire. When heavy rain started to fall, the infantrymen were ordered to retreat. It was a miserable night, with the soldiers waiting in flooded trenches for morning. Ten Americans were dead, and more than three dozen were injured. But much to their surprise, when the sun rose, white flags had replaced the red ones over the fort. The Moros were ready to surrender. Hundreds of their fighters had been killed by the American shells.

This was Kolnitzky's abrupt introduction to the brutal conditions in which he would live for the next two years. Not so much the violence—the Battle of Bayan was by far the worst fighting he would see—but the mud, the heat, and the constant threat of disease. Many more Americans would die in the Philippines from germs than from battle. Malaria, dysentery, typhoid fever, cholera, and smallpox were everywhere, waiting to attack. A few dozen soldiers, like Kolnitzky, would also unknowingly pick up *Mycobacterium leprae* bacilli and bring them home, not discovering for years that they had been infected.

Leprosy was much more common in the Philippines than it was in the United States. At the time, there were an estimated four thousand cases in the island nation, such an alarming number that the Americans running the colonial government were already making plans to isolate the victims. U.S. public health officials used Hawaii's confinement of leprosy patients on the island of Molokai as their model. That effort, started in 1865, had shown questionable success, with hundreds of native Hawaiians misdiagnosed and tragically quarantined. But the idea of segregating leprosy patients had taken hold in the international medical community. The plan for the Philippines was to build a similar colony on the island of Culion, two hundred miles from Manila. There were some leprosy asylums in the Philippines already, but patients generally lived closer to their families and segregation was seldom enforced. U.S. authorities wanted a more "modern" approach as part of their campaign to reshape Philippine civil society in the image of the West.[4]

It did not go well at all. Filipinos with leprosy—like Hawaiians who had the disease—resisted. They understandably did not want to be cut off from family and friends, and they did what they could to avoid being detected. American physician Victor Heiser, who oversaw the project, quickly realized he faced the same challenges Isadore Dyer had confronted in Louisiana. The plan would work best if patients voluntarily agreed to be isolated. "If the work of collecting lepers could have been rushed through with military rigidity, the problem would have been very much simplified," Heiser later wrote. "But it was deemed advisable to precede the collection of the lepers by a campaign of education and thereby secure the cooperation of the public rather than its opposition."[5]

But it was difficult to convince Filipinos to give up their freedom when several prominent physicians continued to insist that leprosy was only a mild threat. Dr. William Henry Welch of Johns Hopkins Hospital called leprosy "practically the least contagious of all the infectious diseases." Dr. William Osler, known as "the Father of Modern Medicine," dismissed fears that the disease would spread as "entirely fanciful." The New York Medical Society declared that leprosy was not contagious at all.[6] Heiser said these doctors were "sentimentalists," who were trying to block "the magnificent hope of the complete eradication of this plague from the face of the earth." Eventually, thousands of Filipinos would be forced to move to Culion, which became known as the Island of the Living Dead.

The debate was almost as fierce back in the United States, where concern about the disease was growing. Louisiana had its Leper Home, but other states dealt with leprosy and other frightful illnesses in a haphazard way, often in response to public hysteria. When a Chinese immigrant died in San Francisco of bubonic plague in 1900, a terrified city cordoned off its Chinatown neighborhood, forcing twenty-five thousand people to stay inside. The quarantine was brief, but it showed the extent to which people would go to protect themselves from disease. U.S. senator George Perkins of California had complained earlier that San Francisco was also caring for a dozen leprosy patients, most of Chinese descent, at the local pest hospital.[7] He called it an "undue burden" on residents and proposed that Congress require all leprosy patients on the mainland to be deported to Hawaii, which had become a U.S. territory in 1898.[8]

Perkins's suggestion was not taken, but the public clearly wanted action. Congress turned to the U.S. Marine Hospital Service, which was responsible for stopping diseases from entering the country. Lawmakers asked the agency, soon to become the Public Health Service, to investigate the extent of leprosy in the United States and to recommend ways to prevent it from spreading. After a yearlong investigation, a panel of three doctors identified only 278 cases in the entire country, although they said there were probably many more. "On account of the loathsome nature of the disease, which has clung to it from antiquity, there is an inclination on the part of the patient himself, as well as upon the part of his family and friends, to conceal the affliction from the public," read the panel's final report.[9]

The Marine Hospital Service recommended that Congress establish a national leprosarium, preferably two of them. It cited numerous experts, including Dr. Dyer, who warned that the disease "seems to be rapidly on the increase."[10] Other witnesses who appeared before the panel said that a national leprosarium was needed to give those with the disease a safe, decent place to live because patients were often shunned by family and friends. One doctor testified that an Indiana man suspected of leprosy had been "lassoed like a wild steer and tied down like a wild beast by the marshal." Two young women believed to have leprosy were driven fifty miles in a wagon to be put on display at a meeting of the Ohio State Medical Association. "When they arrived the cry of 'Unclean! Unclean!' was set up, as it was in the time of Moses," the doctor said, adding that the women had to sleep on the floor of the dissecting room at a medical college because they had nowhere else to stay.[11]

The Marine Hospital Service said the national leprosarium should "be made as attractive as it is possible to make them, so as not to be looked upon as a species of poorhouse or prison by the victims of the disease."[12] But when the House of Representatives started to debate the proposal in 1905, the opposition was overwhelming. No state wanted a leprosy hospital inside its borders. One congressman suggested that the national leprosarium be located in Guam. "I do not know what else Guam is good for," he said.[13] Another lawmaker proposed that the facility be built in the middle of Yellowstone National Park. One newspaper endorsed the plan, arguing that "no possible objection can be heard from the lepers, who are sent to an earthly paradise."[14]

Delegates from the territories of Arizona and New Mexico were especially wary because some had suggested that the dry southwestern climate would be perfect for treating leprosy patients. The two territories wanted to be seen as destinations for those seeking a healthy place to live, not as a dumping ground for society's outcasts. "How would you gentlemen in the States like to have the tinkling bell sounding and the white shroud of the leper stalking through your back yard in the morning, as described in *Ben-Hur*?" asked New Mexico delegate Bernard Rodey of his House colleagues. He said New Mexico would "become the most abhorred and shunned locality we have." Ironically, the territories feared that a leprosarium would discourage wealthy tuberculosis patients from moving to the region to recuperate. Tuberculosis was a far more contagious, prevalent, and dangerous disease, but it did not carry the same stigma.[15] If anything, TB patients were romanticized, as though the disease somehow made them more virtuous and creative.

New Mexico's legislature passed a resolution urging the House to reject any legislation creating a "leper colony" in its territory, "for we consider it an insult that our fair and healthy commonwealth should be chosen by Congress as the abiding place for such unfortunates, with all its attendant evils and miserable repute that such an establishment would entail upon our prosperous and growing territory."[16] Some lawmakers argued that the country had a responsibility to take care of leprosy patients, now that the United States was a world power, and that the disease

was "one of the numerous evils which we have brought upon our-
selves."[17] But the House killed the bill and plans for a national
leprosarium were shelved.[18]

————

As the politicians debated, Sister Beatrice's successor, Sister Benedicta Roach, was trying desperately to keep the patients at the
Louisiana Leper Home comfortable and alive. By early 1902,
twenty-one of them had died from illnesses related to both the disease and the poor living conditions along the Mississippi. In April,
Sister Benedicta curtly notified the board that another name could
be added to the list: "I write to inform you of the death of Clara
Mertz."[19] The woman whose sad fate had led to the creation of the
Louisiana Leper Home was thirty-two years old. When Mertz left
the New Orleans pesthouse for Indian Camp, a reporter had speculated that she would not live long, because she was so ill. But she
had survived there for another eight years. There are no records of
Mertz's time at Carville or how she died.[20]

Sister Benedicta was a strong-willed, no-nonsense woman,
who "didn't believe in enduring anything you didn't have to."[21] She
especially did not like answering to board members who showed
little interest in what was going on at Indian Camp. "Between you
and myself they are a sleepy crowd," she told her mother superior
in Emmitsburg. Sister Benedicta speculated that the men did not
bother to visit because they were too busy with their "sails and
stocks" or because "their wives . . . won't let them come."[22] Her letters to the board were short, businesslike, and often defensive.

Sister Benedicta's relationship with the board did not get off to
a good start. She and Ralph Hopkins, a new doctor hired to treat
the patients, complained to the board in 1902 that the housing was
still inadequate, with two and sometimes three patients crowded
into the small rooms of the wooden cabins. When something broke,

patients were forced to make their own repairs because "outside mechanics will not risk working within the Leper enclosure." Sister Benedicta asked the board why anyone would want to come to the home if conditions did not improve. "Patients, who willingly sought the Home, become discouraged and discontented on viewing the situation to which they have subjected themselves voluntarily," she wrote.[23]

There were now forty patients, only nine more than when the sisters arrived six years earlier. Many were not doing well. Dr. Hopkins presented the board with a sad litany of cases, identified in the public report by number rather than name. Number 1 was a fifty-one-year-old Creole male who had had leprosy for twenty-one years and whose brother, son, and cousin also had the disease, "present condition advanced, treatment chaulmoogra oil, condition unchanged"; Number 21 was a thirty-two-year-old "colored" woman who had been sick for twelve years, "present condition advanced, no treatment, condition unchanged"; Number 59 was a fifty-year-old Irish woman in the early stages of the disease, "refuses treatment, patient insane, unchanged." Eight teenagers lived at the home, including a sixteen-year-old girl, Number 37, who had been ill for eleven years.

Hopkins said that cold temperatures, dampness, and overcrowding threatened to make the patients worse. "There is probably no disease that requires more persistent and thorough treatment, and in the cure of which improper sanitation more greatly interferes," he wrote. Patients with ulcers on their feet had to walk long distances to get their meals or use the outhouse, making it almost impossible for their sores to heal. A broken cistern forced the sisters and patients to haul water hundreds of yards up from the river in wheelbarrows, spilling much of it along the way. "Compelled by law to lead a useless and purposeless life, the unfortunate leper expects . . . that the authorities which compels [*sic*] his isolation, should provide necessities, even the loosest moral code demands," Hopkins wrote. The legislature instead threatened to cut the home's budget, saying that the state was short on funds.[24]

Sister Benedicta complained to the governor, noting that the state seemed to have no problem finding $100,000 for an exhibit at the upcoming World Exposition while its poorest residents were left in need. She then went to New Orleans to plead in person with the Leper Home Board for help. The men initially said there was little they could do, but after she threatened to go public, they agreed to ask for more funding.[25] "It is needless to say that if it be the serious intention of the State to attempt a solution of the leprosy problem, affairs cannot remain in their present condition of uncertainty," the board wrote to the governor and legislature. Something seemed to click. Money was miraculously found to build a new water plant and to replace the old cabins with wooden cottages that included private rooms for the patients. Over the next few years, a rudimentary clinic was constructed, and covered walkways were built so patients could move from one building to the next with greater ease.

Life at the Leper Home improved in other, smaller ways. Beer and fireworks were provided to patients for a Fourth of July celebration. On Easter, they received baskets of colored eggs and treats. For Christmas, there were boxes of candy and fruit, and bigger items such as rocking chairs, bicycles, and musical instruments. Many of the gifts were provided by charitable societies and individuals moved to help the "poor lepers." Sister Benedicta recorded dozens of donations, including cakes, clothing, newspapers, felt slippers, "pretty" cups and saucers, and a "beautiful combination billiard and pool table" from the Crescent City Jockey Club.[26]

But a few trifling amenities did not erase the fact that the patients were confined at a place that was not at all what they had expected. They were not getting cured and, indeed, some were getting sicker and dying. Dyer lamented that the residents were "firmly persuaded that they leave hope behind when they enter the present home."[27]

It was a recipe for resistance. Sister Benedicta reported that some of the younger, healthier patients were becoming insolent. They were sneaking over the wooden fence meant to keep them confined to go drinking or hunting at night. Much to her dismay, some patients also snuck through a fence that separated the men's cabins from the women's. Patient Walter Abrams seemed especially "fond of female company" and upset because "certain pleasures were denied him."[28] Sister Benedicta pleaded with the board to help her impose some rules, such as prohibiting liquor, guns, and the mingling of the sexes. It was enough that the Daughters of Charity had to oversee the patients' medical needs and maintain the property, without having to be disciplinarians too.

Abrams responded by writing directly to the board to defend himself. He complained that he was being treated like a common criminal for violating "outrageous rules" imposed by the sisters. Abrams said his only crime was sitting on a porch talking to a female patient. "It's bad enough we have to be isolated here from the outside world for humanity sake without wanting to take such measures that may make our live [*sic*] more miserable than what it is already," he wrote.[29]

A year later, Abrams ran away, among the first to escape, or "abscond" as it was called at the home. Such escapes threatened to undermine the state plan, as misguided as it was, to control leprosy by isolating the victims. If patients were on the loose, the disease would spread—or so went the common belief. But escapes became more frequent as the patients grew frustrated. A woman named Priscilla ran away repeatedly. She would leave for a few days at a time, then return. Sister Benedicta told the board she suspected that Priscilla was going to a nearby town to get cocaine. Another patient's husband helped his wife escape one evening by sneaking her out in a buggy while the sisters ate dinner.[30]

After Sister Benedicta reported in early 1906 that three women had absconded, the board asked why so many patients, or "inmates" as they were called, were running away. The woman who had begged the board for help could barely contain her anger. She responded with a full-page letter, her frustrations strung together in one long, run-on sentence. The patients were running away, Sister Benedicta furiously wrote, because board members were "lacking in their duty in failing to secure police authority at the home" and had little idea "of the importance of punishing leper patients who persist in absconding."[31] She needed some backup. Shortly after, the board asked the state legislature for $8,000 to build a high steel fence around the patients' quarters.[32] A night watchman was hired, but the patients still managed to abscond.

Iberville Parish residents, who had finally accepted that the home was there to stay, were angered by all the escapes. Louis Carville, the boy who had been disappointed twelve years earlier when ostriches failed to arrive at the property, was now postmaster of the tiny hamlet of Island, where the home was located. (The town's name would soon be changed to Carville to avoid confusion with other towns named Island, and the Leper Home would unofficially assume the name as well.) He and several other prominent parish residents wrote to the board complaining that "inmates of the Leper Home are daily roaming, hunting and trespassing our fields. They have been seen by our citizens roaming through our cotton fields, placing their hands upon cotton balls, which our laborers necessarily must pick, consequently causing them to come in direct contact with disease." The residents had sympathy for the patients, but only so much. "We understand their lot in life at best is indeed sad, but on the other hand can we afford to take chances of contracting said dessease [*sic*]?"[33]

Sister Benedicta had more to worry about than patients touching the neighbors' cotton. One of the patients—"apparently insane," she said—tried to strike a sister with an iron rod and had to be restrained.[34] The same man later entered the dining room with a loaded gun, threatening to kill her. Then four boxes of ammunition were delivered to one patient, who said he needed it for hunting. Sister Benedicta implored the board to do something, noting that some of the male patients had also threatened the night watchman with their guns. "Please send a committee to the Home to take the firearms away from the patients," she wrote.[35] The board responded by warning the patients that if they did not "surrender their arms" to Sister Benedicta, Iberville authorities would be called in to enforce order.[36]

Things were on the verge of falling apart. The patients resented that they were being treated like prisoners. One man protested that he had been threatened with "solitary confinement, a punishment usually doled out to murderers," because he had left the grounds to get something to eat. The patients understandably longed for a normal life. Frustrated, they formed a "patient committee" and in the summer of 1907 came up with what would be the first of many demands. They asked that male and female patients, who were usually kept apart, be allowed to socialize under the massive live oak trees on Sunday afternoons "between the hours of 1 PM and 4 PM, with as many chaperones as you wish to accompany them."[37]

Sister Benedicta denied the request. She insisted that segregation of the sexes was necessary "for sick people sojourning at the Home for medical treatment." Exasperated, the patients asked the board to intervene and to "imagine how greatly these few hours of pleasure will help us to bear the burden of our sorrows, caused by the great affliction for which we are all separated from our homes and families for life. . . . How many sad, dreary, and melancholy hours that they will be turning into joy, sunshine and gladness."[38]

But the board backed Sister Benedicta's decision. It eventually asked the state for more money to build an even taller fence and to hire more guards, noting that "escaping patients have furnished a problem that has puzzled your Board for a number of years."[39] Between 10 and 20 percent of the patients were absconding on average each year. One especially elusive patient ran away more than two dozen times between 1903 and 1920.[40]

It should have come as no surprise that so many patients absconded. The isolation policy was a failure. There was no evidence that the number of leprosy cases in the state was down. If anything, the threat of confinement had forced people to hide their illness, only making the problem worse. It should have been a warning for the rest of the nation.

Chapter 5

"What Have I Got, Doctor—Leprosy?"

JOHN EARLY WAS sick and frustrated. He told his wife, Lottie, as he paced the bedroom floor unable to sleep, that he was overcome by a "terrible sensation." Not so much pain, but agony, like "the fountain of my being is broken up." It was the summer of 1908 and Early had quit his job several weeks earlier at the new Champion fiber mill that stood next to the Pigeon River in Canton, North Carolina, east of the magnificent Smoky Mountains. He found the work dispiriting. The thirty-five-year-old complained that men at the mill were churned up and spewed out like the wood they were supposed to be turning into paper and pulp. Early's job was tending massive tanks of hot, acid-like black ash, a by-product of the process. He said the ash left his skin covered in cankerous sores, poisoned his blood, and made his hands and feet swell. He had had enough.[1]

With one young child and a second one on the way, Early was desperate for money. After talking it over with his wife, he boarded a train for Washington, DC, to file a pension claim with the army.

He had contracted malaria while serving in the Spanish-American War, first in Cuba and then in the Philippines. That should be good for something. When Early arrived in the nation's capital, he rented a room at a Salvation Army boardinghouse on Pennsylvania Avenue, two blocks from the U.S. Capitol, a building whose chambers he would rattle in the years to come. Now, he was simply a supplicant looking for government help.

Early wasn't a big man—about five-foot-eight—but he was lean and taut, with the muscles and chiseled look of someone who had spent long hours doing hard, physical work—chopping wood, plowing dirt, toiling in construction, anything to survive. He had grown up poor in the mountains of North Carolina, which produced a bitterness that cut deep into him like a gorge. Early resented that his parents had to rent their tiny cabin from a wealthier landowner. He resented the snubs of students at the small college he had attended near his home. He resented that he'd had to do janitorial work to pay his tuition. He especially resented when he had to drop out of school for lack of funds and get a job helping to build the largest private home in America, the Versailles-like Biltmore mansion in nearby Asheville. It was being constructed for George Vanderbilt, scion of the wealthy Vanderbilt family, with 250 rooms and sumptuous gardens. Early was bitter as he lugged hundred-pound bags of cement for a meager $1.12 a day, thinking how just one of the mansion's many marble columns could easily pay for his education. "What's the use?" he wondered of his life. Early's path could not have been more different from that of Isadore Dyer, who at the same time was building his medical career in Louisiana after studying at Yale and Tulane. The two men had no idea how their lives would eventually intersect in pursuit of a similar goal, and how the poor North Carolinian would succeed where Dyer had failed.

Early had more immediate concerns as he waited for word

on his pension. His skin itched and burned, and his forehead was swollen and covered with bumps, so he summoned a doctor to the boardinghouse. When the doctor examined his face and seemed confused, Early joked, "What have I got, doctor? Leprosy?" The doctor knew that Early had been a soldier in the Philippines, where leprosy was endemic, and took the question much more seriously than Early intended. He called the city health inspector, William C. Fowler, to the boardinghouse for a second opinion. Fowler, too, was suspicious when he saw Early's face, so the two doctors went for additional help, discreetly locking the visitor in his room as they left. Soon after, a local pathologist came and took a sample of Early's skin to be tested for the *Mycobacterium leprae* bacillus.[2] Just to be safe, the health officials packed up the startled patient, his belongings, and his bedding, and had him taken to an isolated spot along the east branch of the Potomac River, an area of the city set aside for the poor and unwanted. Early slept that night in the back of an ambulance, parked near the local jail, an asylum, and the paupers' cemetery. The next day he was moved to an eight-by-ten-foot white tent by the river and two guards were posted outside to make sure he did not escape. Inside the tent, Early found a cot, a table and chair, and cooking utensils to use while he waited.[3]

Early received the official test results, along with everyone else in the city, in an article on the front page of the Sunday newspaper: "Leprosy in the District: Officers of Health Department Make Discovery," the headline read.[4] Alarm spread through the city and beyond. District health officials assured residents there was little to fear. The army's acting surgeon general, Colonel Valery Harvard, said the belief "that leprosy is so easily transmitted is a rich and foolish statement." He insisted the disease was "only slightly" contagious.[5]

But the health officials' actions belied their words. If the visitor posed no threat, why had he been whisked away to the river? Rip-

ples of alarm followed every step Early had taken on his journey
north. Residents wondered where he had been and what he had
touched. Newspapers speculated that he had been in contact with
"hundreds of people." The story became front-page news across
the nation; a real live "leper" was confined in the nation's capital.
Curiosity seekers soon came to the Potomac by the hundreds to
catch a glimpse of Early in his tent, as the guards warned them to
keep their distance. Some of the gawkers came with home reme-
dies they believed would get rid of the disease. One man carried
a box of what looked like axle grease to be rubbed on the lips and
gums, declaring that this was the cure for leprosy.[6] A visiting evan-
gelist told Christians that their prayers were Early's only surefire
path to salvation. Meanwhile, North Carolina officials refused to
let Early return to their state. They said he was not their responsibility, since he was diagnosed in Washington and had likely contracted the disease while serving in the U.S. Army. The district
was stuck with him.

Early was resigned to his fate. To him, this was another unfortunate blow for a poor boy from the mountains. As the chaos
swirled about him, he sat tall and serene on a wooden chair outside
his tent, wearing a straw hat, jacket, and tie. He passed his time by
reading the Bible and answering questions that reporters shouted
at him from afar. Early told them his main wish was to be reunited
with his pregnant wife and their eleven-month-old son. Lottie had
taken a train up from North Carolina with her mother and child as
soon as she heard the news, but health officials would not allow her
to get close to her husband. They warned that, if she did, she would
lose custody of both her son and her yet-to-be-born child. Lottie
rented a nearby cottage, waiting for some resolution.

She and John were bound by their deep religious faith. They
had met at a Salvation Army service in upstate New York, when
John was still in the military, at what he called a low point in

his life, "drinking, whoring, gambling, carousing." The Salvation Army proved true to its name, saving him and setting him off on a new path with the "wistful, sweet-faced girl" who became his wife.[7] Now here they were in Washington, trying to keep that faith alive. Lottie went to John's tent each night at dusk, stopping ten feet away. Under a guard's watchful eye, the couple recited John's favorite psalm as the sun set: "I will lift up mine eyes unto the hills, from whence cometh my help."[8]

The Earlys found the arrangement on the Potomac unsatisfactory, to say the least. John complained that Lottie and their son were stuck in a "small lonely shack of a cottage" while he was confined to a tent, "smelling sewage, fighting mosquitos, heat and cold." Health officials wrestled for days over how to deliver the $165 pension check that John had finally been granted. Lottie needed the money now more than ever, but no one wanted to touch the voucher that John was required to sign. Finally, someone came up with a creative, if awkward, solution. The voucher was placed in a yellow envelope with two open slits exposing the places where John needed to sign his name, so he could do so without touching the paper. A health official, a doctor, two guards, several newspapermen, and Lottie were all at the tent to witness the momentous event. After the voucher was signed, the health officer removed it from the envelope, which he then proceeded to burn. District residents were assured that the voucher itself would be fumigated before it was stored in the pension office. No safety measure was too small when it came to leprosy, which only encouraged the public perception that there was something dreadful to fear.[9]

Four months after Early was first confined, his second son was born, and he was still in the tent. Health officials had no idea what to do with him, but they knew they had to do something as the temperature began to drop. In December, they finally agreed that John could leave the tent and move into a nearby brick house with his wife, although they were still not allowed to touch each other. To make sure they didn't, a brick wall was built down the middle, dividing the house in half. John had to live on one side, while his wife, children, and mother-in-law lived on the other. John and Lottie communicated through the wall, tapping out messages. On many nights, they sang hymns together as John played his mandolin on his side of the wall and Lottie played a small Salvation Army organ on hers. Sometimes she went into the yard and held the baby up outside John's window so he could see his new son. A guard was on duty at all times to make sure no one violated the rules.

It was an absurd arrangement. Early's quarantine on the banks of the Potomac made it increasingly clear that the United States was ill-prepared to handle a disease that so alarmed the public. Louisiana had its Leper Home, and San Francisco and Massachusetts had smaller facilities where leprosy patients were confined. But that was it. Each time someone was suspected of having the disease, it threatened to become a national health scare, with sometimes fatal outcomes. On the same day the Early story broke, newspapers reported that a California woman had gone "crazy" when she learned she had leprosy. Her husband, a Civil War general, had snuck her out of the Los Angeles County hospital's contagious ward so they could flee to Mexico. But authorities caught the couple in Arizona and confined them to a tent in Tombstone. As state officials debated what to do next, the woman's elderly husband died. So they packed her into a train car and sent her back to Los Angeles, where she was strapped to an iron cot in the county hospital. She died soon after, but not before a nurse who had worked with leprosy patients in India suggested that the patient be chloroformed and put out of her misery.[10] The papers called the woman's treatment "tragic and pitiable." But it was not that uncommon.[11]

Two years earlier, the fate of another leprosy patient had also gripped the nation. A twenty-one-year-old immigrant named George Rashid had decided to return home to Syria after being diagnosed with the disease in Elkins, West Virginia. Money was raised—it's unclear if by friends or by residents eager to see him leave—to buy Rashid a train ticket to New York City so he could take a ship home. But the train ride turned out to be far more perilous than the disease.[12] When word got out that a "leper" was on a passenger train headed to Maryland, authorities tried to stop him at the border. Rashid got off before they could apprehend him, but he was eventually found and put in a boxcar on a freight train bound for New York. The story of his flight quickly hit the newspapers, rousing the public's anxiety and morbid fascination. Government officials went on high alert. The Washington, DC, health department assured district residents that it had deployed sentries to the borders in case Rashid headed their way. Reporters tracked his every move. When Rashid's train stopped briefly in Maryland, the young man reportedly emerged "half starved" from the boxcar and "inspired fear in the breasts of all who knew of his presence." Some of those who came out to see Rashid tried to help the desperate man by throwing food at him and placing water on the ground nearby, before running away.[13]

When Rashid finally reached Philadelphia, city health officials refused to let him go any farther. The young man had to wait in the boxcar while the authorities figured out what to do next. "His stay in the city lasted eight hours, which was eight hours longer than the health authorities wanted him," reported the *Philadelphia Inquirer*.[14] Eventually, they ordered the rail company to take Rashid back to West Virginia, but the train was stopped again as it approached Baltimore. Maryland health authorities did not want Rashid either but were sympathetic and hoped to find some way to get him to New York—where officials were willing to accept him—and out of the country. For the next eight days, Rashid was confined in the boxcar while authorities haggled over his fate. When he left the train at one point looking for food, the *Baltimore Sun* said nearby residents panicked, calling their children into their houses and bolting the doors.[15]

Finally, Maryland health officials decided they had no choice but to send the young man back to West Virginia. To avoid frightening the public, they secretly brought Rashid to the Baltimore train station late at night in a disguise. Maryland's top health official, John Fulton, accompanied him to the state border, where he informed West Virginia officials that the Syrian was headed their way. The authorities removed Rashid when the train reached the small town of Pickens, West Virginia, and isolated him in the woods in a tent—and later a shack. Local residents were furious and rumors began to circulate that Rashid would be lynched if he stayed. The state tried to get the federal government to take him off their hands, with no luck. A man hired to nurse Rashid fled after he was threatened by a mob when he went into town for supplies.[16]

Within three months of his arrival in Pickens, Rashid was dead. A doctor who had cared for him said he died of heart failure and questioned whether the young man had even had leprosy. Still, just to be safe, Rashid's shack was burned to the ground and the boxcar he rode in was destroyed. Workers on the Baltimore & Ohio Railroad had threatened to go on strike if they were forced to go near it again.[17]

Rashid's treatment was widely condemned by physicians, national health experts, and the press, even though many of them had, in their own way, added to the hysteria. The *Washington Post* complained about "childish panic" over leprosy and said that "germ theory has simply run amuck tainting persons whose judgements on other matters are sober and accurate."[18] Fulton, the Maryland health official, complained about Congress's failure the year before to create a national leprosarium where those with the disease could get proper care. He said maybe Rashid's case would finally inspire lawmakers to act.[19] U.S. surgeon general Walter Wyman said the "absurd alarm" over Rashid had prevented the case from being handled appropriately.[20] Even Isadore Dyer weighed in. He said the Syrian had been treated with "criminal inhumanity" and concluded that he died from "chagrin and neglect," rather than leprosy.[21]

Some of the fear and confusion was understandable. Not only were health authorities still divided over the seriousness of the threat, no one knew how the disease was spread and there was no known cure. Even if the chance of contagion was slight, it was a risk many were unwilling to take.

Two years after Rashid's tragic death, John Early's case was a reminder that little had changed. He sat imprisoned in his divided brick house as public health authorities continued to wring their hands. Some suggested that Early be sent to the colony in Hawaii or maybe to the Philippines. Others questioned whether he really had the disease at all or, if he did, whether he needed to be confined. The result was that Early was stuck where he was, his hair growing longer by the day because no one was willing to cut it. Eventually, his mother-in-law was allowed to do the job.[22]

In the spring of 1909, nine months after Early was first quarantined, a prominent New York dermatologist came to Washington at Lottie's request to examine her husband. Dr. L. Duncan Bulkley was skeptical that Early actually had leprosy. Bulkley spent hours examining him, pricking his skin dozens of times to check for numbness. He also took skin samples to test for presence of the bacillus. Bulkley concluded after a week that Early did not have leprosy and that his skin problems—which had all but cleared up by then—were more likely the result of his work at the pulp plant. Bulkley pressed district health authorities to let him take

Early to New York City for further examination at the Skin and Cancer Hospital, where he worked, and where Isadore Dyer had also interned.[23] Washington, DC, officials were not convinced that Bulkley's diagnosis was correct, but they were happy to get Early off their hands. It was costing the district thousands of dollars to keep him confined.

Late on the night of July 3—almost a year after he first arrived in Washington—a carriage picked Early up and took him to Union Station. Newspaper reporters who came to cover his departure said he looked the "picture of health," wearing a gray suit with white shirt, dark tie, and new patent leather shoes. Early pulled himself into a baggage car that had been set aside for him and two acquaintances who had agreed to join him for the overnight trip. Early was optimistic that his troubles might be nearing the end. "Now, I feel that I will return to work and be able to feel that life is worth living," he told the reporters. "When I reach New York I expect I will soon be lost sight of and be able to settle down to business."[24]

The train arrived in Jersey City, New Jersey, the following morning. Early and his companions quickly jumped out of the baggage car and caught a ferry to New York, joining the other passengers on deck to enjoy a cool breeze as they crossed the Hudson River to lower Manhattan.[25] It was Independence Day, the Fourth of July, and Early looked forward to having some independence of his own to celebrate. Within days he did. Doctors at the New York hospital declared Early free of the disease and allowed him to leave. Even if he had leprosy, New York authorities did not believe he should be confined. Unlike officials in other states, they did not consider the disease to be a serious threat, one of those inconsistencies that kept the public so confused.

By coincidence, the city was dealing with another high-profile health scare at the time. Mary Mallon, an Irish cook, had been quarantined at the city's pesthouse on North Brother Island because she was suspected of spreading typhoid fever in the homes of prominent citizens, where she worked. The week that Early arrived, Typhoid Mary, as she was known, was fighting for her freedom and had complained in court that she was being treated "like a leper." The irony was not lost on the editors of the *Brooklyn Daily Eagle*. "It is to be hoped that Early, the alleged leper, will not join forces with Typhoid Mary and write a book about doctors they have met," they wrote.[26]

Understandably tired of the notoriety he'd lived in for the past year, Early hoped to enjoy his newfound freedom in obscurity. He was soon joined by Lottie and the children in Brooklyn, where they lived under assumed names. But their stay was cut short. Newspapers reported that Gerhard Hansen, the Norwegian doctor who had discovered the leprosy bacillus, had examined some of Early's skin tissue and concluded that the North Carolinian did indeed have the dread disease.[27] Early and his family fled Brooklyn and moved to a farm in Virginia. But Early was still desperate for money, and three months later he made the mistake of returning to Washington to claim $196 in uncollected pension payments. He was immediately arrested and placed once more under quarantine. After several days of legal wrangling Early was again put in a baggage car and sent to New York, where he was once again declared disease-free and released.[28] One prosecutor called the case "a sort of farce." "It appears that John R. Early is officially a leper in the District of Columbia, but is not in New York," wrote the *Washington Times*.[29]

The Earlys continued to ricochet around the country, trying desperately to escape the stigma that seemed to follow them everywhere. They eventually landed in Southern California, where Early worked on ranches and farms until his health began to deteriorate in 1911. He later revealed that one of his New York doctors visited him in California and admitted that he had made a mistake with the diagnosis. Early did have leprosy.[30] Discouraged, the Earlys—who now had a third son—packed up and moved to Tacoma, Washington, looking for new opportunities and anonymity. But when he reapplied for his military pension, John admitted to Tacoma health authorities that he had leprosy. They said he could continue to live on his property as long as he stayed in a cabin fenced off from the rest of the family. But when word got out, the neighbors reacted with predictable dismay. Parents took their children out of school, and about a hundred residents gathered at the local Methodist church and signed a petition urging that Early be sent away.[31] "They ought to put a millstone around his neck and throw him in the ocean," one woman said.[32]

A frustrated Lottie decided to seek help right from the top and wrote a letter asking then-president William Howard Taft to intervene. Lottie told the president that she needed her husband's pension money to "save the little home for our children's sake and [it] would be a very small sum to the government compared with what it will mean to us and our little ones."[33] Taft was already under pressure from veterans' groups to do something about Early. It was unseemly for the government to be hounding a man for a disease he had likely contracted while serving his country in the military. Taft's solution was almost Solomonic. He said that Early could get his monthly pension of $30, and an additional $65 a month, if he moved to a quarantine station on Puget Sound to care for a sailor who was confined there with leprosy. Early agreed, and in March 1912 he moved to the Diamond Point Quarantine Station. His family stayed behind. The strain had become too much on the marriage. Lottie would later allege that Early was physically abusive to both her and the children and they were soon divorced.[34]

For two years, Early cared for several men with leprosy who had ended up at the station, but he eventually became restless. The disease was beginning to cause him intense pain and sensitivity in his head and eyes, which can happen when the bacteria attack crucial nerves. He was also despondent over the loss of his family and freedom. Early began to hatch a plan. One morning in May of 1914, he served the other patients breakfast, slipped off the grounds, and caught a boat ride across Puget Sound to Canada, where he boarded an eastbound train.[35] His destination was the city he had agreed never to reenter, Washington, DC. Early's plan was to make a case for himself—and the nation's other leprosy victims—once and for all.

Chapter 6

Finding a Home

Moving people with leprosy from one place to another was a challenge. Sometimes more challenging than finding a place to take them. How could patients be transported without risking public health? Or causing a panic? An individual with leprosy was generally not allowed to cross state lines without the written permission of each state's health authority. If one state objected, the patient was stuck. But some doctors thought the restrictions were excessive, even counterproductive, and the rules were inconsistently applied. When John Early took that first train to New York City, he and his traveling companions were forbidden from getting off at the Jersey City terminal with the rest of the passengers, because the train company feared Early might contaminate the others. Instead, the three men got off the train as it sat nearby in the rail yard, walked into the station, got in line, and purchased ferry tickets along with everyone else. They then joined the people they had been isolated from on the train for the trip across the Hudson.[1] It was one of the many contradictions in how he was treated that drove Early—some thought literally—crazy.

It was fitting, then, that Early booked the finest transportation he could find to make his way back east from Puget Sound. "I had my face set like a flint on the very important city, Washington, D.C," he wrote.[2] He was on a mission to prove that the public had an irrational, often cruel reaction to his disease and that he and other victims suffered needlessly as a result. Early had concluded, after years of being chased from one place to another, that a national leprosarium was needed to protect people like him. So he had saved up his pension money while living at the quarantine station and purchased a first-class ticket for a Pullman car on the Canadian Pacific line. The accommodations were probably the nicest Early had ever had. He said his fellow passengers were "elite and congenial" and included Canada's former governor general and his family. Early took his meals in the elegant dining car, with its cushioned seats and fine linen, as he watched the dramatic scenery flash by. He was so drawn by its beauty that at one point he considered getting off and losing himself in the Canadian wilderness. But he decided his trip was too important to abandon.

Early took his time reaching Washington, so he could interact with as many people as possible—breathing their air, rubbing their arms, shaking their hands, resting in their chairs. He stopped for a few days in New York City, where he strolled along Manhattan's crowded streets, attended a Broadway show, and enjoyed a baseball doubleheader between the Yankees and the Philadelphia Athletics. He then continued on to Washington, where he booked a room under an assumed name at one of the city's most exclusive hotels, the Shoreham, a block north of the White House, across Lafayette Square. The hotel had recently been renovated, its grand lobby painted a muted brown with gold trim. President Woodrow Wilson had been a guest at the hotel the year before while awaiting his inauguration. Vice President Thomas Marshall and his wife, as well as several senators and ambassadors, now made the Shoreham their home. Early mingled with them all, at one point riding in the elevator with the vice president.[3] The fugitive leprosy patient could not have picked a more prestigious place to make his point. He spent a couple of days visiting the sights, including the Washington Monument, soaking in his last minutes of freedom.[4]

Almost three weeks after setting off from Puget Sound, Early was ready to go public. He alerted a couple of newspaper reporters that he was back in town and invited them to join him in his hotel room. He then called the health department to report his return. The newspapermen were there to witness as William Fowler, the official who had ordered Early's confinement years earlier, walked in followed by an agitated hotel manager and house detective. "Hello, Doctor Fowler," said Early. Fowler was more resigned than surprised. "I thought I recognized your voice over the telephone," he said. The health official, after hearing about Early's escape from the quarantine station, had suspected that he might be headed back to the nation's capital, and was prepared. He took Early down to a waiting car and drove him to the same house by the Potomac River that he had shared five years earlier with his family. Only now, the windows were secured with iron bars. The room at the Shoreham Hotel was promptly sealed off and fumigated.[5]

Early had finally accepted his fate. He said the old John Early was "dead to the world. . . . From now on I am willing to be isolated, to have the warning bell of the 'unclean' rung as I approach, to feel that men shrink from me with the world-old fear of the terrible disease that has been laid upon me, but I want my appeal to be heard." Those who knew Early from before thought his condition had worsened. He was no longer the picture of health as he had been when he left Washington five years earlier for New York. His forehead was deeply furrowed, his nose and ears were bloated, and

his hands were swollen. "I know I am a leper now," he told reporters. "But I want my case to serve as a great national example and
bring about the proper treatment of the unfortunates."

Early had calculated every step of his trip to make the biggest
splash. He might have been crazy, as some believed, but he was
extremely astute at manipulating public opinion. "I knew that if
I mingled among the well-to-do and the rich and exposed them to
contagion that they would arise out of self-protection and further
my plan of a national home," he said. "That is why I chose the Pullman cars, why I slept at the best hotels, ate in the best restaurants.
No one cares what happens to the poor. If I had kept to the slum
the agitation would have been light."[6]

His scheme worked. Early's dramatic escape and reemergence
became front-page news across the country. "Suspected Leper in
Washington Hotel Brings Panic," reported the *Salt Lake Telegram*;
"A Leper Invades," blared the *Muskogee Times-Democrat*; "Supposed
Leper Found in Vice-President's Hotel," read the *Harrisburg Telegraph*. But the *Washington Times* admonished the public for overre-
acting. "The case of John Early, leper, has been an amazing series
of demonstrations that American civilization is yet afflicted with
a good deal of the barbarism of the Middle Ages. Early has been
handled in the District of Columbia, in the State of Washington,
and elsewhere throughout the country, in a way that shows how
liable the public is to fall into panic over that which it does not
understand," the paper wrote. "Nobody wants him, and nobody,
in the face of the strange, medieval terror inspired by his disease,
seems concerned whether he shall be given civilized treatment."[7]

No one was more disturbed by Early's return than district
health officials. They thought they had gotten rid of one of their
most difficult patients once and for all. Now, he was back, challenging them as the entire nation looked on. Lawmakers on Capitol Hill were furious. Representative John Raker of California

called Early's escape from the West Coast quarantine station "worse than turning loose a band of murderers." Within hours of the news that he had returned to the capital, three bills were introduced on the House floor—one to establish a national leprosarium, another requiring that Americans with leprosy be sent to Hawaii, a third calling for a board to determine whether Early actually had the disease. None of the bills passed, but the push for a national leprosarium had gained new momentum.[8]

Isadore Dyer and others used Early's case to press for the kind of action that had eluded lawmakers so far. Both the country and patients needed protection, they argued. "While leprosy is slowly contagious and probably mildly contagious, its usual horrors argue the danger of neglect. With probably 500 known cases today, how many will there be in ten years, if there is no control?" asked Dyer at a meeting of the American Medical Association. William Rucker, the assistant surgeon general, warned the same group that a "veritable leprophobia" had gripped the nation. "Let a man be marked as a leper and he becomes a pariah, an outcast from society, to be hounded from place to place, to be locked in a lonely, often filthy, building, there to be viewed at a distance by the more intrepid as some wild and dangerous animal."[9] Still, the United States wasn't as bad as some places. Only two years earlier, thirty-nine men, women, and children with leprosy were driven into a pit by soldiers near the city of Nanning in southern China, and burned alive as "the rejected of heaven and useless encumbrances of the earth."[10] A ten-dollar bounty was offered to those who caught anyone else there with the disease.[11] There was a long way to go before the world would accept this widely loathed illness as relatively benign.

Finally, in 1915, the House agreed to establish a national leprosy hospital, but only after adopting an amendment requiring that the facility be located, in the words of one lawmaker, "out in the wild somewhere, where nobody lives within a radius of many miles and where nobody ever will live."[12]

The Senate held hearings on the bill the following February, almost two years after Early's stunning return to Washington. He remained confined in the lonely house on the eastern branch of the Potomac, becoming increasingly depressed. Louisiana senator Joseph E. Ransdell, chairman of the Committee on Public Health and National Quarantine, which was holding the hearings, went to see Early the evening before they were set to begin. The next day, Ransdell told the committee that Early, a man "who has gone through terrible sufferings," said that "he and every other poor leper in the United States, in his judgment, would be delighted to go to a national home, where they would have a great many comforts and at least companionship."[13]

Fowler, the district health official, was called to testify. He told the committee that Early was under arrest for entering the district "without a permit" while suffering from leprosy. Fowler assured the lawmakers that Early would have a hard time escaping. There were bars on his windows and door, and the house was surrounded by an eight-foot-high barbed-wire fence. "You are now treating him practically as a wild animal?" one of the senators asked. "Practically, I am afraid," Fowler responded. "We have to in order to keep him."[14]

Dyer was also a witness at the hearings. He had never meet Early but knew that the recalcitrant veteran had handed him the most powerful argument yet for a national leprosarium. Dyer shifted his position slightly, though, telling senators that public fear of the "leper" was perhaps the main reason the federal government should open a facility. "He is discriminated against in all public places, to the end that he becomes an outcast and an object of horror in spite of the fact that the danger of contagion from him is about 1 to 100 as compared with the tubercular patient," Dyer testified. "He not only bears all the burdens of his disease, but he also bears the burdens of centuries of opprobrium which makes him psychopathically different from a patient suffering from any other disease. For that reason they need just that much more care." In other words, Dyer was now arguing that isolation was needed more because of social prejudice than to protect society from a dangerous disease.[15]

In January of 1917, Congress finally agreed to spend $250,000 to set up a national leprosarium. The law did not require leprosy patients to be confined there but gave state health officials the power to decide, something almost all of them would use to send these unwanted residents away.

Despite widespread support, the law took another four years to put into effect. The country was preoccupied with a war in Europe, and, as expected, it was not easy finding a site for the new hospital. The U.S. surgeon general wanted to locate the facility on Penikese Island, seven miles off the coast of Massachusetts in Buzzards Bay, where that state already housed a dozen leprosy patients. But complaints by nearby residents forced him to abandon the idea.[16] Similar protests erupted over proposed sites in West Virginia and elsewhere. When states were asked for suggestions on where they thought the home should be located, they inevitably pointed somewhere else. West Virginia thought California would be a good place to put it. Alabama suggested Texas. North Dakota recommended Colorado.[17] The Public Health Service eventually purchased two islands off Cedar Key in Florida and was ready to start building the facility there when Florida businesses and politicians got wind of the plan. They launched a vigorous campaign against the federal home, arguing that it would devastate the state's economy by discouraging tourism and destroying the market for its valuable citrus crops. One resident grumbled that no one would buy fish caught in nearby waters "with the sewage from this colony emptying into them."[18]

At one point during the search, Victor Heiser, the American doctor who had set up the Culion colony in the Philippines and was now back home, visited Gulfport, Mississippi, for unrelated business. When he got off the train, he was met by an angry mob. Heiser could smell hot tar and saw someone in the crowd holding a bag of feathers. "This is the guy!" one man shouted. "We're going to make an example of you," cried another. Rumors had been circulating that a government official was coming to check out a proposed site for the national leprosarium on a nearby island and the crowd had mistaken Heiser for the official. He was saved when someone shouted that it looked like they had the wrong man. "This guy hasn't any whiskers," he called out, and Heiser was allowed to pass. It turned out that the person the mob was looking for was hiding in his hotel. The clerk told Heiser that the hotel managers planned to smuggle the man out on the first train the next morning.[19] The Gulfport site, like all the others, was crossed off the list.

A few officials had suggested using the Louisiana Leper Home in Carville for the national hospital, but the idea was quickly dismissed as impractical. The location was too remote and the climate unsuitable for those with leprosy. Still, the patients at Carville followed the developments closely and eleven of them ran away in the first half of 1919. Sister Benedicta speculated that it was because they had heard rumors the government might build the new leprosarium on a remote island. They did not want to be forced to move there and end up even more isolated than they already were.[20]

———

By the summer of 1918, John Early had been confined in the house near the Potomac for four years. He was extremely lonely and frustrated, and his physical condition was getting worse. He was tormented by shooting pain in his nerves and took morphine to ease his suffering. He had become gaunt and weak. Some days, he could do little except lie in bed or sit up and "peer out through my screened and bar-darkened windows, across the monotonous mud-flats of the Potomac" and "listen to the incessant shrieks of the locomotive whistles and jarring, rumbling thunder of the almost constant stream of freight trains crossing the long bridge not more than a thousand feet away." Early often slept only a few hours a night. "I could neither read, think or pray with any composure. So depleting and devastating to my being had it become that it seemed God had entirely forsaken me," he later wrote. If the leprosy didn't get him, the isolation would.[21]

Early was desperate to get out. The thought of another winter confined in the dismal house by himself was too much to bear.[22] In the early morning hours of September 16—when the night guard was apparently dozing—Early sawed off the bars on his window, squeezed out, and ran to a hole in the barbed-wire fence that surrounded the house. Officials speculated that Early probably had an outside helper who provided him with the saw. The fugitive patient caught a cab to a nearby town, slept for a few hours, and stopped at three separate doctors' offices to pick up an ample supply of morphine before boarding a train for North Carolina. Along the way, he also got a copy of the evening newspaper.[23] Below a banner headline that read, "Germans Continue to Retreat," was a smaller one: "John Early, Leper, Again Flees from Prison Home." A side-bar urged readers to "Watch for This Man!"—"John Early, leper. Five feet seven or eight inches. Weighs about 100 pounds. Has peculiar leprosy nodule on cheek. Walks with difficulty, owing to swollen feet. Hair reddish. Cheek bones very prominent. Last seen wearing gray cap, gray suit and tan shoes."[24] No one on the train seemed to notice or care.

Authorities eventually tracked Early down at his family's home in Tryon, North Carolina, but once again, with no national lepro-sarium, they were uncertain what to do. The District of Columbia did not want him back, and he did not want to return. North Carolina did not want him either. Finally, Louisiana officials agreed to take Early at the Leper Home, even though the facility was supposed to be reserved for state residents. They would make an exception for the man now known as the nation's "most famous leper." Early was taken to Carville under armed guard, and on November 16, 1918—more than ten years after asking that fateful question, "What have I got, doctor?"—John Early became patient Number 306.

Ninety men and women were living at the Louisiana Leper Home when Early arrived. Conditions had slowly improved over the previous two decades, and Sister Benedicta called it a "magical change" when the candles and kerosene lamps they used were finally replaced with electric lights.[25] She told the board in 1918 that she had an "optimistic view of the future," in part because twenty patients had recently been discharged as "cured"—although they were more likely experiencing temporary improvements in their conditions, or spontaneous remission, which sometimes occurred. Many of these patients ended up returning later, as sick as before. Still, the discharges were seen as a sign that patients had benefited from the care they received at the home. "Each of these cures is as the star of hope to every inmate of the home, bringing a degree of happiness and contentment into lives which would otherwise be strangers to all but gloom," wrote Sister Benedicta.[26] The Daughter of Charity who had run the home since 1901 was nearing retirement and had recently loosened some of her strictest rules, which helped to boost morale. Male and female patients who were related—either as siblings or as parent and child—were now allowed to visit each other once or twice a week in a designated area. It wasn't much, but it was something.[27]

Early was not impressed. "Did not take me more than five min-utes in the door of the 'Carville Leper Home' to learn that I would have to clash with the mathematical, meticulous creed of the nuns in charge. In face [*sic*], I had a strong prompting before I reached it, that I would not fit into its groove," he wrote.[28] Early made it clear that he disliked living under the supervision of such a "hard-boiled character" as Sister Benedicta and it wasn't long before he was encouraging his fellow patients to agitate for their rights. In March of 1920, Willard Centlivre, a World War I veteran, fol-lowed Early's advice and escaped from Carville to go to Washing-ton, DC, to air his grievances. Centlivre told authorities that his family was destitute because of his confinement and he needed a pension. He was promptly taken to Early's old house by the river until he could be returned to Louisiana.

Centlivre then shocked health officials with some disturbing news. He warned that Early was planning to have all the patients at Carville escape and come to Washington to press their demands for better care. He told a Louisiana congressman who came to visit him that the nation's leprosy victims were an organized fra-ternity and could wield a lot of power. "U.S. Officials Unearth Secret Plan for Big Parade of Lepers in Capital," warned a head-line in the *Washington Times*. "Centlivre is said to be an advance agent for the 'army of lepers' being mobilized for the march on the Capitol."[29] For several days, the city was on high alert, bracing for the possible invasion of hundreds of leprosy patients. One offi-cial assured the public that "the leprosarium will notify us imme-diately of any escapes and we in turn will post lookouts in all Southern states in an effort to catch them before they gain any headway."[30] It turned out that the threatened march was a hoax, but the panic it caused reminded the country that it had yet to set up the long-awaited national leprosarium.[31]

Frustrated that they were unable to find a more suitable site, federal health officials finally decided to take over the Louisiana Leper Home. There were still concerns about sending patients to such a hostile environment. The property was infested with disease-carrying insects, water moccasins, and rattlesnakes, and was vulnerable to flooding. But it seemed the best, if only, choice. The residents of Iberville Parish had long ago accepted the home as part of the community. Many of them even worked there or made a living selling it food and other supplies. The state was also happy to unload the facility on the federal government, because the Leper Home was expensive to run. It turned out to be a good deal for the federal government. The home came with a committed and experienced staff, the Daughters of Charity, and plenty of space to expand. The price was also hard to beat—$35,000 for everything.

On January 3, 1921—seven years after Early's sensational return to the capital—the Louisiana Leper Home became U.S. Marine Hospital Number 66, under control of the Public Health Service. Isadore Dyer was not there for the occasion. He had died four months earlier of heart failure and did not see his life's dream come true. But John Early was there when three Daughters of Charity helped to unfurl the American flag. He watched as the flag, whipped about by the river breeze, rose up the pole in front of the mansion, where it would stay for the next seventy-eight years.

Early would not stay. He would soon flee the hospital—the first of many escapes by the disgruntled vet.

Chapter 7

Ripped Apart

A 1917 PHOTO shows Terville and Lucie Landry of New Iberia, Louisiana, sitting straight and proud, amid the fruits of their marriage. Terville wears a suit and bow tie; Lucie has on a homespun dress and rimless glasses, her hair pulled back from her face. The couple is surrounded by their five children, all looking healthy and robust. The youngest, Amelie, leans gently against her father's thigh. Albert, the next youngest, sits at his mother's knee, her hand resting on his shoulder. Standing behind them are the three oldest, in their teens and early twenties—Norbert, Marie, and Edmond. Norbert wears a hint of a smile, as though he can hardly contain his joy. No one in the photo knows that at this very moment, *Mycobacterium leprae* is attacking at least one, if not more, of their bodies. Over the next six decades, all five Landry siblings will end up at Carville. All of them will die there, not from leprosy but from other illnesses such as tuberculosis, kidney disease, and heart failure.[1]

Hansen's disease is not hereditary. Nor is it contracted through sexual intercourse or childbirth. But it is not unusual for a parent and child, or multiple siblings, to get the disease. One ten-year-old patient at the Louisiana Leper Home, patient Number 201, was listed as the brother of patients "69, 104, 220, 221, 222, 223, and 246."[2] Most people are naturally immune to the disease, but relatives are more likely to share the rare genetic susceptibility. Family members also tend to live close together, over long periods of time, making it easier for the germ to move from one to another, perhaps with a cough or a sneeze, or a child's runny nose. But the disease spreads so slowly, so invisibly, that no one realizes the damage has been done until it's too late.

That's what happened to the Landrys, who fell one after the other: first Norbert, then Edmond, then little Amelie, followed later by Albert and Marie. For most of a fifty-eight-year stretch, from 1919 through 1977, one or another Landry would be a patient at Carville. Together, they would witness the hospital's growth from an isolated, ill-equipped asylum into a first-class medical institution. They would see the patient population evolve from a body of hopeless victims into a potent political force. But the disease and its stigma would also tear apart family relationships and leave a lasting mark on descendants, who would learn many years later that they were known in their hometown as the "leper Landrys." Edmond's wife and children, like Morris Koll's, would keep his illness a secret for decades.

The opening of the nation's first leprosarium meant that hundreds, if not thousands, of American families were about to be ripped apart. While the patients were clearly the victims, so too were the parents, children, spouses, and siblings who were left behind. Secrecy, scorn, and shame would shadow their lives. Financial ruin would often be around the corner. The emotional scars would last forever. All in the name of protecting the public from a mildly contagious disease that people feared more for the image it evoked than for any actual danger it posed.

Some families, like the Landrys, had it worse than others. Norbert was the first to be diagnosed, two years after the family portrait was taken. He was twenty-four years old, just back from France, where he had served in the army during the Great War. He was engaged to be married, thrilled to be home, and eager to get on with his life. But three months after his return, a doctor gave Norbert a diagnosis that hit with the force of an enemy shell. He told the young veteran that his blemishes were a sign of leprosy and encouraged him to go some eighty miles east to what was then still the Louisiana Leper Home. The doctor assured Norbert that he would be treated well there and might even be cured, a farfetched possibility that the young man optimistically embraced. Expecting to return home soon, Norbert did what many patients did. He asked his parents not to let anyone know where he was. He assumed an alias—James Jackson—to protect himself and his family from humiliation and scorn.

Norbert's family was extremely supportive. They treated the young man more like a college student away from home for the very first time than like someone fighting a loathsome disease. They visited him at Carville and sent food and candy and even a little dog named Zip to keep him company. Norbert was eager to get better and faithfully employed the main treatment options he had at the time—chaulmoogra oil, good hygiene, and prayer. He was deeply religious, a strong believer in the power of faith, and his condition a year later was listed as "markedly improved."[3] Norbert tried to keep busy, attending church each day, hunting (Sister Benedicta was now retired and so, too, it seems, were some of her rules), painting, and watching the movies shown at the home each week. Still, he told his family it was a "lonesome" place.[4] Norbert hadn't been there long when his fiancée broke off their engagement, the first hint that his life would never return to normal.

Norbert had high expectations when the federal government

swooped in and took over in 1921. He wrote his brother Edmond in March that U.S. health officials were waiting for thirteen new patients to arrive from Penikese Island in Massachusetts and were "rushing to build some Temporary Houses to receive many more."[5] The government's plan was to eventually have enough housing for four hundred or more patients from around the country. Norbert said he was encouraged by the new medical officer in charge, Dr. Oswald Denney, who had run the Culion colony in the Philippines for four years. Denney told the patients that the Red Cross planned to send "14 phonographs, one player piano and two motion picture machines" for them to enjoy. Norbert said even the food was better under federal control, with eggs every day, milk three times a day, potatoes, and even fish and ice cream. "I tell you that this little Dr. is putting this place up to date, and that is a great thing for us. We are surely thankful for that. But I myself I hope that I don't have to stay here much longer," he wrote to his brother.[6] Norbert lived at Carville for three more years, until he died of tuberculosis, just shy of his twenty-ninth birthday.

Edmond was devastated by his younger brother's death, and had an additional reason to grieve. He knew by then that he, too, had leprosy, and it was getting worse. Edmond was thirty-three years old and serious, with thinning hair and growing respon-sibility. He was married to Claire Gragnon, a young woman he had met after she missed a train and he kept her company while she waited for another. A photo taken a few years later shows the young couple sitting on the porch of a house in New Iberia, gleam-ing with joy at their firstborn child, a chubby baby girl propped up on Edmond's lap, her round tongue popping out like a ball. It was the picture of domestic contentment, a young, healthy family with a promising future. But two years later, shortly after a son was born, that happiness was shattered. Edmond's doctor told him he likely had leprosy, something Edmond may have suspected. He had been bothered for years by some numbness on the skin near his ankle. But his doctor was more progressive than most and said he would not report the case to state health officials because it was in its early stages and extremely mild. He told Edmond that he could continue to work at his bookkeeping job and live at home while his condition was monitored.

After a year, Edmond's symptoms grew worse. His hands and legs started to weaken and the doctor said he should stop working, although he could stay at home as long as he limited his contact with others. It was better than going to Carville, but far from desirable. Edmond's wife, Claire, had seen what the disease had done to her brother-in-law and was terrified that her husband might infect her and their two young children. She made Edmond agree to live "as sister and brother" and refrain from sexual relations. The children could visit their father in his room, but they were not allowed to touch him. The painful arrangement lasted for a year and a half, until shortly after Norbert's death, when Edmond finally agreed that he, too, should move to Carville. Technically, he volunteered to go, but his doctor said that if Edmond did not willingly commit himself, he would be taken there in shackles.[7] On October 10, 1924, Edmond kissed his family goodbye, a rare act of intimacy, and drove with his father and uncle to the place where his brother had recently died. His children were ages five and three. Edmond would never live with them again.

As the Landrys' tragedy unfolded, Morris Kolnitzky was back home in New Haven, building a business and raising a family. He had returned from the Philippines in 1904 and gone to work for a grocer. But he soon became restless and went out on his own, opening one meat market, then another, his business growing along with the city. Morris was heavier than he had been in the army, but still strong, and took up amateur boxing in what little spare time he could find. He had an aggressive, no-nonsense air, as did the woman he married, Dora Brower, a Jewish immigrant from Poland. Dora had a pile of lush brown hair that she kept pinned on top of her head; a white, egg-shaped face; and thick, dark brows over her equally dark eyes. They were a formidable pair, working their way along the classic immigrant path to success. They were no longer Kolnitzkys. Morris had shortened his name to the more American-sounding "Koll." They had three children, Leo, Helen, and Harold.[8] By 1922, the future looked bright. Koll's latest meat store was in a prime location, next to the gothic enclave of Yale University. When the shop first opened, the man who served as governor general of the Philippines while Koll was there, former president Taft, was a law professor at the university. The famously rotund Taft would sometimes stop by on his way home from work to pick up a bologna sandwich.

Koll might have seen the sensational news stories about John Early, a fellow veteran who had also served in the Philippines. It's even possible he discussed the bizarre case with Taft, who had helped Early in response to his wife Lottie's appeal. Even so, Koll was certainly too busy to worry about something as remote as leprosy. Like Norbert Landry, he had no reason to be concerned when he went to see a doctor for what seemed like a relatively minor complaint. The thirty-seven-year-old butcher had noticed that his legs would sometimes swell above his ankles, hardly unusual for someone who was overweight and spent hours on his feet. But his fingers and one of his toes also felt numb, a potential hazard for someone who butchered meat for a living.

Koll was stunned by the diagnosis. The doctor believed that the veteran had probably picked up leprosy in the Philippines eighteen years before. He also had some other devastating news for his patient. The federal government had recently opened a leprosarium in Louisiana, and under Connecticut law, the doctor was obligated to report Koll's case to the health department. Koll would likely be sent to Carville—more than a thousand miles away—and confined there for the rest of his life.

Koll's first thought was suicide. "I wanted to do away with myself, to end it all."[9] It was a common response for those diagnosed with leprosy. Two years earlier, Norbert Landry had written to Edmond about a patient at the Leper Home "who was so disgusted and worried over his family that he took some Poison tablets. He said he was better off dead than to worry this way. But he didn't succeed." The man threw up the pills and survived.[10] The Daughters of Charity cited numerous other suicide attempts over the years. "Sad news!" one wrote in 1936. "Patient who was taken by the Immigration Officers on January 9th for deportation to Patras, Greece, shot himself on board the steamship in New York City." And in 1942: "A terrible thing has happened on this Good Friday. A patient, Mike, a Greek, commits suicide by swallowing lysol. Could not be saved."[11]

Koll came home that night distraught. But as he looked in on his two youngest children, who were sound asleep—Harold and Helen, ages two and four—he decided against taking his life. The doctor had given him another, seemingly farfetched, option. He told Koll that neighboring New York had different rules than other states. Health officials there did not think leprosy was contagious or that patients should be isolated unless they had open skin lesions, which Koll did not. He could move there and keep his freedom, but he had to act quickly before his case was reported. Koll packed his things and departed that night, leaving his business and family behind. Dora would manage the New Haven market while Morris established himself in New York. She and the children would join him later and, hopefully, their nightmare would be over.

Patients came to the new national leprosarium from near and far, and from all walks of life, taken from those they loved and deprived of their liberty. Federal health officials had hoped to make the hospital so attractive that victims would willingly come to the secluded spot. But, as Isadore Dyer had discovered before them, it was a difficult sell. Few patients wanted to leave their families for the rest of their lives. For every person diagnosed with the disease, an estimated four or more remained undetected, misdiagnosed, or living in secret like Morris Koll. A year after the hospital opened, the assistant surgeon general announced that there were "1,200 lepers at large" and he wanted to be given the authority to round them up.[12]

Many of the earliest patients to arrive at Carville had been languishing in hospital isolation wards around the country, and were now gathered up like pieces of bruised fruit to be tossed away. With the establishment of a national leprosarium, state health authorities could wipe their hands of the responsibility. The first patients included people like twenty-two-year-old Hazel Deuser of St. Louis, who learned she had leprosy the same way John Early did—from a newspaper headline. "Girl Leper Found in St. Louis," it read. Deuser, a single mother with a new baby, was confined at the local hospital for several months until it was time for her and two other St. Louis patients to be moved down south. One was a Chinese immigrant, who had been confined for more than fifteen years and was described in the local newspaper as "hopelessly insane." The three patients were put in a Pullman car, joining twelve others who had been picked up in St. Paul, Minneapolis, Milwaukee, and Chicago. This pitiful band of patients was accompanied by a doctor, two nurses, and two orderlies, who wore rubber gloves when handling their charges. The public was assured that for much of the time the health workers would be separated from the patients by a curtain soaked in disinfectant.[13]

Since children were not allowed at the leprosarium unless they, too, had leprosy, Deuser was forced to leave her six-month-old daughter behind with her parents. The child was eventually told that her mother had been hospitalized for a nervous breakdown, which was more socially acceptable than admitting she had leprosy.[14] Deuser would not see her daughter again until she escaped from Carville five years later.

———

Unlike his brother, Edmond Landry was not at all optimistic that he would ever get better. He tried to make as much as he could of his new life at Carville, knowing he most likely would die there. He assumed an alias, Gabe Michael, and set up what was sardonically called the What Cheer Club. It distributed proceeds from a patient-run canteen—where small personal items were sold, like tobacco, stockings, and gum—to those at the hospital who were blind and indigent. Edmond tried to stay positive but his letters home were packed with sorrow. He missed the foods, like gumbo, crawfish, and cherry bounce, that were staples of his former life. He repeatedly asked family members to send fresh-picked pecans that he could share with the other patients. Edmond was heartbroken that he could not watch his children grow, and he desperately longed for his wife. Claire came to visit, but not often enough, he complained. The children were not allowed to visit him at all.

Edmond became increasingly depressed. In the spring of 1927, heavy rains swelled the Mississippi to historic levels, threatening communities all along its banks. The patients and staff at Carville worked furiously, piling up sandbags to reinforce the small earthen levee that protected the property, which was low and flat and easily flooded. Edmond warned Claire that he doubted the patients would be saved if disaster hit. "If the thing gets worse and breaks will you all—you and the folks—come to get me and my gang," he pleaded. "You know I never liked levees anyway and now being a 'leper' I wonder just how much rescue help would come to us in distress and as close as I can figure it the majority will say let them drown, it's good riddance." A barge had been positioned on the river to evacuate the leprosarium if necessary, but Edmond believed it would be used to save only the staff.[15] One of the Daughters of Charity who worked at Carville said the intention was to evacuate everyone, but even she doubted the plan would work. "There were handicapped people who couldn't walk and some were blind, and if they would have had to get them out there—I don't think they would have made it," she said.[16] Fortunately, the Carville levees held and the patients survived one of the nation's worst natural disasters. But the Great Mississippi Flood of 1927 was a stark reminder of how isolated and vulnerable they were.

Edmond watched with sorrow as more patients arrived, day after day, many of them pitifully young. They included two brothers, ages eleven and thirteen, from Newark, New Jersey. After they were diagnosed, Frank and Hale George—as they were identified in newspapers across the country—were immediately removed from their school. The building was fumigated, and after the teachers threatened to resign, all fifteen hundred textbooks used at the school were burned.[17] Soon after, a twenty-year-old woman named Rita was brought to Carville by her father, who did not tell her she had leprosy until they arrived at the gate. When he returned to their home about thirty miles away, he informed everyone that his daughter had died, and she never saw him again.[18] There was also Buddy, an orphan from New York, who was brought to the leprosarium in 1928 at the age of five. The little boy was so upset when

he arrived that he threw an orange at one of the sisters, knock-
ing off her white cornette.[19] Buddy was soon joined by seven-year-
old Oscar Dempster. Oscar had been taken to a hospital in New
Orleans for a foot injury, but doctors there determined he had leprosy, wrapped him up in a sheet, and took him to Carville. Oscar
was more fortunate than some of the other children. His older sister
was already a patient there and in some ways Carville was better
than home, where his widowed father had seven other children to
care for. Oscar put on his cowboy hat and rode his tricycle up and
down the long walkways that connected the buildings like a giant
web.[20] He lived there until he was ninety-one.

Edmond's sorrow slowly turned to anger. He was increasingly
upset about how leprosy patients were treated by society. He did
not believe that he, or any of the others, was a threat to public
health. Edmond was especially disturbed that his wife, Claire,
visited so infrequently and that, when she did, she refused to get
physically close. In June of 1928, his pent-up frustration exploded
in an eighteen-page single-spaced typewritten letter, one tightly
wound sentence after another. "Dear Claire: For nearly four long
years I have begged you to treat me better than you have," he
began, pleading with her to visit him at least once a month "as my
wife." He said if she refused, "I will then know that I belong in
the 'land of the unburied dead.'" Edmond insisted that Claire had
nothing to fear, that if she were prone to leprosy she would have
contracted it already after seven years of living together. He complained that leprosy patients were treated "like cast away rubbish,"
while those with far more dangerous diseases—such as tuberculosis and syphilis—were allowed to be free. "It is the thought of all
these things and the realization of how the public does not care to
have us out of here, whether parolees or absconders, that all but
runs us nuts," he wrote. It was an extraordinary letter for a man
who prided himself on being rational, responsible, and faithful to

his family. The threads of his life were unraveling, as it became clear that his fate was likely to be the same as his brother's.

Edmond's physical condition was deteriorating. He had severe headaches, nerve pain, and swollen legs and glands, none of which was helped by the chaulmoogra oil he took for relief. Shortly before writing to Claire, he sent a desperate note to the U.S. Veterans Bureau asking what would happen to his insurance and benefits if he should escape from Carville, or even die. The bureau responded that all payments to his family would stop. Someone at the Veterans Bureau was so alarmed by the tone of Edmond's letter that he forwarded it to Dr. Denney, Carville's chief medical officer, noting that it appeared "it is the intention of the veteran to either elope from your institution, or destroy himself." Edmond apparently decided that he could not risk leaving his family destitute, so he did neither, although he threatened to run away if his wife did not begin to treat him better. Claire continued to visit him at Carville—although it's unclear how often she came or how physically close she was—until he died in 1932 from kidney failure, a common side effect of leprosy.

Edmond Landry's children had only faint memories of their father. Patients from Louisiana, Texas, and Mississippi were sometimes allowed short, restricted visits home, and Edmond went to New Iberia twice to see his ailing mother. "He came under armed guard—and that's something I've never forgiven them for, and I never will," his daughter, Leonide Landry Manes, known as Teenie, recalled decades later.[21] She remembered playing across the street from her home when a car drove up with her father and two officers "with their leggings and their khaki pants and their stiff military round brim caps and the gun on the side. . . . It scared me to death," she said.[22] The little girl thought her father was a prisoner.

———

In 1927, there were three hundred people confined at the federal leprosarium, and a nineteen-year-old debutante from New Orleans was about to join their ranks. Edwina Parra led a charmed life. She was engaged to a handsome medical student. She had a secretarial job that she loved. She spent evenings going to the theater and dances. Edwina, by all accounts, was lovely and refined, a young woman who never had a hair out of place or uttered an impolite word. Her family members called her a "little priss" because of the way she fussed over her clothes and loved to take long, luxurious baths. Edwina was the oldest of five children, part of a large, close-knit Catholic family from what she called "old French New Orleans" stock.

The family's togetherness was on full display that Christmas, as everyone gathered in the grand Garden District home of her grandparents, sharing rich food and singing Christmas carols around the piano. After dinner, there was a poker game for the men, fireworks for the children, and skits performed for all to enjoy. Edwina barely noticed when one of her uncles, a doctor, stopped by and told her father that he needed to speak with him right away. But she recalled later that her uncle seemed unusually sad when he kissed her goodbye.

Edwina had recently consulted one of her uncle's colleagues, a dermatologist, about a few rose-colored spots on her thigh that wouldn't go away. The spots seemed little more than a nuisance, a minor problem easily resolved, as every problem in her life to this point had been. But her uncle told her father that they were anything but minor; Edwina had leprosy. Her parents were stunned and decided not to tell their daughter until they got a second opinion. They took her to another doctor, who confirmed the diagnosis and advised them to send Edwina away at once, before she infected anyone, especially her four younger siblings.

Edwina knew that something was amiss, but, in a sign of the

times, she was too dutiful to insist that her parents tell her what was going on. Her fiancé, Robert, finally offered to be the one to tell her. The young couple had plans that night to attend a dance at the Orleans Club on St. Charles Avenue. He brought Edwina pink camellias to match her short lace dress. He told her how beautiful she looked, but she could sense that something was wrong. They left the dance early, and instead of stopping at a café for beignets and café au lait, as they usually did, they went straight to her house. In the parlor, Robert wrapped his arms around Edwina and told her what the doctor had said. The young woman was horrified. Leprosy was a disease that belonged in biblical times, not in twentieth-century New Orleans, and certainly not for her, a vivacious teenager with her whole life before her. Robert assured Edwina that she would have to go to a hospital near Baton Rouge only until she was cured. He said it would not take long and that he would be waiting for her when she returned.

Two weeks later, Edwina, her mother, and Robert drove along the long gravel road that hugged the Mississippi on the way to Carville. Her parents were adamant that no one should find out the real reason why Edwina was leaving home so suddenly. Friends and family were told that Edwina had contracted tuberculosis and would be away for a while. "So began an elaborate network of duplicity under which I was to cower for the rest of my life," she would later write.[23]

Carville looked nothing like what Edwina had imagined. She had expected dark, moss-covered stone buildings that resembled tombs, with patients slowly moving about shrouded in rags. Instead, she was struck by the beautiful oak trees, the grand mansion, and the cozy-looking patient cottages. Under federal control, Carville was starting to look more like a country retreat than a hospital, with one exception. The property was still surrounded by a high fence topped with barbed wire.

Edwina's mother rang the bell at the mansion and they were soon greeted by one of the Daughters of Charity. The government had decided to keep the women on as nurses, in part because it was difficult to find anyone else willing to do the job. Sister Catherine Sullivan hugged and kissed the young woman and, to help ease her fears, suggested that they go to the chapel to pray. Sister Catherine assured Edwina's mother, a devout Catholic, that her daughter was there on a mission and that all would turn out well in the end. "Mama clung to the prophetic words, praying they might someday come true," wrote Edwina, who admitted that she did the same.

Like other new patients, Edwina Parra assumed an alias. She became Betty Parker—later Betty Martin, after she married another patient and took his last name, which was also an alias. Sister Catherine took Betty to the cottage where she would live with eleven other women, but Betty did not expect to be there for long. She was determined to get better quickly and return to her charmed life in New Orleans, maybe in six months or so. But like many of her fellow patients, she would end up spending much of the rest of her life at Carville.

Chapter 8

"Nun Nurses"

Sister Hilary Ross talked like a gangster. Not because of the words she used but how she spoke them, out of one side of her mouth. The other side of her face had become partially paralyzed when surgery for an infection behind one of her ears went bad. Two follow-up surgeries failed to fix the problem, which was complicated by bouts of typhoid fever and pneumonia. As a result, Sister Hilary suffered from constant headaches. "I have never had what you might call a well day since," she said later. But her misfortune landed her at Carville, where she worked for thirty-seven years and did medical research that would have a profound impact on hundreds of thousands of lives. She could relate to the patients' pain and disabilities, although she dismissed her own as inconsequential, saying that "one learns to live with one's ailments."[1] For many years, the federal government paid her a dollar a year—quite the bargain, considering what she accomplished.

Over the course of Carville's history, 116 sisters worked there as nurses, pharmacists, biochemists, dietitians, and physical therapists. They would prove to be some of the patients' strongest allies in their fight for more freedom and rights. But the relationship was bumpy at times, producing deep divisions at what was supposed to be a nonsectarian government medical facility. The sisters' presence once again tied the dreaded disease to religious faith. The decision by Dr. Denney, Carville's top medical officer, to keep the Daughters of Charity on as civil-service employees proved to be one of his most controversial. But he needed their help. Six sisters were at Carville when the federal government took over, all of them experienced nurses. Denney doubted he could find anyone else who was as skilled and would be willing to move to rural Louisiana to work with leprosy patients.

Sister Hilary came, in 1922, because the federal government needed a pharmacist for the new leprosarium. She had studied pharmacy at the University of Wisconsin after the Daughters of Charity moved her out of the nursing program because of her botched surgery. She was smart, methodical, and focused—a perfect candidate for the job. She was also tough and had a survivor's mentality, helpful attributes for those working at the remote facility. One colleague called her "the hard-boiled type," although another described her as "a soft-boiled egg in a hard-boiled shell." She stood about five-foot-six, with rimless glasses perched on her beak-like nose. Despite the facial paralysis, she spoke loudly and intently, often grabbing the arm of the person she was addressing to make sure her message was heard. "Regularity and exactitude were a part of her," one sister said, adding that while Sister Hilary "never indulged in jokes herself" she would laugh at the jokes of others.[2]

Sister Hilary was an unlikely candidate for the sisterhood. She had been raised a Protestant and discovered Catholicism while learning to make corsets at a lingerie shop. She was born Mary Helen Ross in Berkeley, California, in 1893, one of seven children.

She was only twelve years old when her father drowned in San Francisco Bay, leaving her mother to raise the children on her own. Less than five months later, tragedy hit again. San Francisco was devastated by a massive earthquake that forced Mary Helen to flee with her mother and siblings as flames approached their house on Telegraph Hill. They had no time to take much more than the clothes on their backs, as they ran with thousands of others down to the wharf to catch a ferry to Berkeley and emergency shelter. It was a chaotic scene and she saw "many sad sights other than the destruction—women were hysterical and there was much weeping and lamenting." She knew what it meant to lose everything.

The Ross family was now homeless and Mary Helen soon had to find work. She ended up as an apprentice at D. Samuels Lace House, one of the most exclusive women's shops in San Francisco, where she made friends with another young woman. That woman was a devout Catholic, who attended Mass every day at noon. One day, she invited Mary Helen to accompany her. Mary Helen had been baptized Episcopalian but agreed to go, and was soon attracted to the rigors of Catholicism, which gave structure to her otherwise unsettled life. She eventually decided to convert and then to join the sisterhood, over the strong objections of her mother. Mary Helen was especially attracted to the Daughters of Charity, who were known for their care of the poor and disadvantaged. She later said her decision was sealed when she saw the image of a sister's white cornette on the host she received at Communion one day—an unusual admission for a woman who was so grounded in science that she would one day become an internationally known expert on Hansen's disease.

It must have been a shock for the twenty-nine-year-old sister to arrive in the Deep South on a hot summer day, straight from the relative chill of Milwaukee, where she'd been living. The humid Louisiana air was unlike anything she had ever experienced before. Conditions at the leprosy hospital, although slowly improving with the recent federal takeover, were still primitive. Her pharmacy turned out to be a small space in one of the old cottages, which doubled as a doctor's office and operating room. The only equipment she was given to provide medication for the more than ninety patients now living there was a scale for weighing drugs.[3] She had to mix all the medications by hand, relying on lots of elbow grease to blend the ingredients.

Sister Hilary soon discovered just how isolated she and the patients were from good medical care. One night shortly after her arrival, she felt a pain on her right side. By 1 a.m. it was so intense, she went to the room of her superior, Sister Catherine Sullivan, for help, but seeing her sound asleep, Sister Hilary decided not to disturb her. By 4 a.m. she could wait no longer. Sister Catherine immediately realized that the new sister had appendicitis and needed to be rushed to the closest hospital, which was in New Orleans. They had to take a five-hour trip in an old army ambulance along bumpy, mostly unpaved roads. By the time they reached the hospital, Sister Hilary's appendix had burst; it took her months to recover.[4] When Sister Catherine later asked why she hadn't alerted her sooner, Sister Hilary responded sheepishly that she did not want to bother her because she was sleeping. "What do you think I would be doing at that time of night? Making biscuits?" Sister Catherine responded.[5]

Sister Hilary would prove far less timid in the pharmacy, and she immediately got down to work. Ironically, the establishment of a national leprosarium had taken away some of the incentive to find a cure and better medical treatment for those with Hansen's disease. With the patients off the streets, they were considered less of a threat to public health. Out of sight, they were also out of mind. There were other, far more dangerous, diseases, such as polio and influenza, attracting medical research and dollars. A polio epidemic in 1916 had killed 6,000 Americans and paralyzed thousands more. Two years later, the flu killed 675,000 people in the United States, and 50 million worldwide. Leprosy was a distant, relatively minor concern, although thousands of Americans were still believed to have the disease.

As they had for decades, Carville patients relied on chaulmoogra oil as their primary medication, even though it made many feel sick to their stomachs. Sister Hilary decided that she wanted to fix that.[6] She tried combining the chaulmoogra oil with cocoa and flavored syrups to see if she could make the medicine more palatable. She experimented with more than fifty combinations—each of which she tasted herself. But nothing seemed to work. Patients were still throwing up the medication. Sister Hilary finally put the oil in gelatin capsules that slowly dissolved in the patients' digestive tracts, easing the impact. It was a minor improvement, but one the patients appreciated. An alternative treatment was to have the oil injected, sometimes into their buttocks, which patients complained was extremely painful.

Most Carville residents believed the chaulmoogra oil was worthless, but they had few options. The oil had been used in Asia for centuries to treat leprosy. According to folklore, a Burmese prince was cured after the gods directed him to eat the seeds of a related tree.[7] While some people insisted that the oil helped heal leprous skin lesions, Norway's Gerhard Hansen believed the medicine was worthless.[8] By the 1920s, most patients at Carville treated the oil as a joke, another sign of their sorry state—stuck in the backwaters of medical research, along with everything else. The only advantage was that patients were allowed an unlimited supply of the pills. One man routinely collected a large number of them, admitting later that he used the oil to grease his hair.[9]

While Sister Hilary was busy trying to find better ways to care for the patients' physical well-being, another Daughter of Charity was focused on their mental and spiritual health. Sister Catherine Sullivan was the woman who wrapped her arms around Betty Parker (the former Edwina Parra) when she arrived and assured the young woman she had nothing to fear. Sister Catherine came to Carville in March of 1916, when it was still the Louisiana Leper Home, and was well aware that those who were admitted seldom left. But the sister was an optimist, outgoing and full of life, with a perpetual smile that produced prominent dimples beneath her plum-shaped cheeks. She was determined that the patients should not lose hope and knew that besides fighting germs she had to help them fight despair.

Sister Catherine was born Margaret Madeleine Sullivan in 1886, in Texarkana, Texas. She was an avid reader and was deeply influenced by the writings of Charles Dickens, whose destitute characters gave voice to social injustice. The Daughters of Charity seemed a good choice for her to right some of the wrongs that were prevalent in America in the early twentieth century. The order sent her first to work as a nurse at St. Mary's Hospital in Milwaukee and then across the street to St. Rose's orphanage, where she taught girls from troubled homes. One former student wrote Sister Catherine years later that as she stood on a bridge contemplating suicide, "suddenly, just as I was about to spring, your face came before me, just as I had seen it so many times in the asylum back at Saint Rose." The woman decided to not jump rather than disappoint the sister who had helped her as a child.[10] The orphanage was a perfect fit for Sister Catherine and she was ready to settle in.

But the Daughters of Charity urgently needed another nurse at the Louisiana Leper Home, and she was selected to go. One of her earliest duties there was to greet and admit new patients, an important job since she was their first contact in what could be a frightening place. One day, a few years after she began working at Carville, Sister Catherine was in her office on the first floor of the mansion when she heard the sound of horses' hooves and iron wheels crunching along the gravel road outside. Two new patients were expected that day, a woman in her early fifties and her adult daughter, and they had come with the older woman's son. Sister Catherine went out to greet them at the front gate since patients were not allowed on the staff side of the property. When the son declared, "I have brought my mother and my sister," Sister Catherine immediately thought of the story of *Ben-Hur* and how the hero's sister and mother were exiled from Jerusalem because they had leprosy. "I felt angry panic rising within me. Was our 20th century no different from the 1st?" she later wrote. "Had we stood still thru the centuries?"[11]

The women's story was a common one. They had gone to the doctor to have what they thought would be a routine examination of minor blemishes and were shocked when he ordered them to go to Carville immediately. The son begged for more time so that his mother and sister could get their affairs in order, but the doctor replied, "This is Tuesday. You can have until Friday."

Sister Catherine climbed into the carriage to show the women to their new lodgings in the cottages behind the mansion. "I'll ride down with you," she said, trying to sound cheerful. She asked the son if he would like to come along to see where his mother and sister would "be living for awhile," even though she knew that "awhile" probably meant forever. The carriage rolled down the dirt road alongside a low privet hedge that divided the staff side from the patient's side. As they passed through an opening in the hedge, Sister Catherine looked away from the others, aware of the fate that awaited them. "With one turn of the wheel they had passed into a different world—and only I knew it," she later said.

Sister Catherine became increasingly disturbed by the patients' isolation from the rest of the world, exiled for nothing more than carrying a mildly contagious germ. As she stood near

the patients' cottages one day looking toward the river, she realized that the view was blocked by a seven-foot-high wall of weeds.
Patients could not even see the road they had used to get to Carville. "Only a road, yes, but it led back and out, and to my mind it
stood for all the roads of the world which the patients have a right
to travel—unhindered and untrammeled. How could they keep the
goal in mind, if the very road were lost to view?"[12] To her, the wall
of weeds symbolized all the prejudices, ignorance, and unjustified
fears that prevented the patients from leading normal lives. In a
sudden rage, she grabbed a cane knife and began hacking away.
Within minutes, several patients ran out, insisting that it was no
job for a sister and they would take over. They thought she was
trying to clear land for a garden. Sister Catherine responded that
the patients should go get their own knives and they would hack
down the wall together.[13]

The sisters and the patients knew that in many ways they were
allies—deserted and forgotten together. "There is a splendid feeling of camaraderie between the patients and the personnel," said
Sister Catherine. "Quite as there would be between a hospital
unit and the boys in the front line trenches." In fact, patients at
Carville would soon find themselves on the front lines fighting for
their rights, and Sister Catherine was among those who would
nudge them along. She believed that leprosy was a social disease
more than anything else and that the victims needed to speak up for
themselves. When a reporter asked decades later what her biggest
impression was from working at Carville, Sister Catherine looked
around at what had become a modern hospital, but where patients
were still confined. "My outstanding impression is that mercy is
no substitute for justice."[14]

Although stern in appearance, and sometimes in reality, the
Daughters of Charity were some of the patients' closest friends and
confidantes. But the arrangement was highly unusual for a fed-

eral facility. The patients who came to the Louisiana Leper Home from around the state were overwhelmingly Catholic. Now that it was a national institution, there were also Protestants, Jews, Buddhists, and atheists, some of whom bristled at having caretakers who answered to both the government and God. Involvement in religious activities at the hospital was supposed to be voluntary, but non-Catholic patients started to complain that some of the sisters were proselytizing on the sly, and even out in the open.

Not surprisingly, John Early was among the most vocal critics. He was a Protestant—a religious fanatic to some—but he strongly believed that religion and medicine needed to be kept apart. He refused to call any of the Daughters of Charity "Sister." Instead, he referred to them as "nun nurses." Or "Nun Mary" and "Nun Catherine."[15] Early complained that the women were trying to convert patients to Catholicism and in some cases were succeeding. "I don't blame them if they do make every mother's son and daughter of us Catholics," he railed. "But I do blame the federal government for promoting this advantage. And if the federal government cannot 'nurse' its leprosarium . . . independent of organized religious charity, then it should admit its defeat, pull up the U.S. stakes, take down the golden flag and turn the 'Leper Home' back to Louisiana and the supervision of the Catholic Sisters."[16]

Early was not the only disgruntled patient. When he was not on the lam, he would gather with some of the other male patients in a makeshift clubhouse they had built at the back of the property so they could have some privacy and independence. One observer said it looked like a battleship galley inside, with a gas range, aluminum utensils, and a large radio set in the corner. Most of the members were veterans like Early, and they would spend evenings together, drinking, smoking, and building up rage at their sad lot in life. In 1924, he helped to turn that rage against the Daughters of Charity. He and thirty other patients signed a petition that read, "We, the undersigned, protest their employment in the government's institution, and request their removal, and that trained nurses be employed in their stead as a preventative of proselytizing and religious favoritism that is obtaining under their (Sisters') nursing."[17]

The controversy simmered for months but finally came to a head in the spring of 1926, after patients complained about the two chaplains who worked at Carville. The Catholic chaplain had annoyed some of the Protestant patients by refusing to allow a military ceremony to be included in the funeral Mass for one of the veterans. A Catholic patient then came to blows with the Protestant chaplain over his presence in the cafeteria, which patients considered off-limits to outsiders. Word of the unrest reached Washington and the Public Health Service sent one of its surgeons, John McMullen, to find out what was going on. After a quick inquiry, McMullen reported that religious disagreements at the hospital were "deplorable" and getting out of hand. "There is an unrest and high tension among the patients which cannot continue," he said. "Numbers of the patients stated that if present conditions continue, which they referred to as a war, they would be obliged to abscond."[18]

In late May, McMullen, Assistant Surgeon General William Terriberry, and another doctor were sent to Carville to investigate further and to find the source of the religious unrest. Over two days, they took testimony from Dr. Denney, both chaplains, two sisters, and more than twenty residents. It was soon clear that there was a sharp divide between the Protestant minority at Carville and the Catholic majority. The Protestants complained that the sisters sometimes placed religious items, such as medals, in patients' rooms, even as they lay dying. They also said the sisters discriminated against non-Catholic patients when providing nursing care. "The Catholics are the dominating power. They like to be bosses," testified patient Charley Brown.

The head of the Catholic faction was a patient named Billy Lee, who did indeed like to be in charge. He came from a political family in New Orleans and operated like a ward boss at Carville, doling out favors to supporters and friends when he was put in charge of the patient canteen.[19] Lee defended the sisters and blamed "crazy" John Early for the turmoil. "If you move the Sisters you will ruin the morale of this camp," Lee told the investigators. Patient David Palmer also blamed the unruly veterans for the unrest and asked Denney "whether this is a hospital or a battlefield." The investigators were given a petition, signed by more than a hundred Catholic patients, calling for the sisters to be retained.[20]

The health service officials then interviewed the two Daughters of Charity, who had a different take altogether. They blamed the disturbances on the patients' general dissatisfaction with being confined. Sister Martha Lawlor, who was chief nurse at the time, said it "boiled down that the patients feel they are certainly prisoners here" and were resentful. Sister Catherine told the investigators that she believed the controversy was not about religion at all. "The patients' antagonism and quarrels are by no means confined to religious topics. They cannot have a ball game, they cannot have a tennis game, they cannot have a moving picture show on any other than the regular night but there must be a fuss and fight about it," she said. "You would get the same answers you are going to get about religion if you asked them about ball games or tennis courts." She recommended that any sister found proselytizing be dismissed.

Denney also told the investigators that those who opposed the sisters were "a small, decidedly biased group." There were now thirteen Daughters of Charity at the hospital and he defended them as hardworking and loyal employees. Denney insisted that the government would be hard-pressed to find anyone else to do their jobs. "The manifestations of leprosy in these infirmary cases is so repugnant and so repulsive that only women of considerable stamina could continue in such work," he told the panel.

Assistant Surgeon General Terriberry agreed. He concluded that there was indeed some proselytizing by the sisters. "There have been unseemly occurrences relative to the fighting over dying lepers as to which side would get them and bury them," he wrote in the investigators' final report. He said there was no question that some sisters had placed "emblems of the Catholic faith in the rooms, and even on the bodies of helpless or dying Protestant patients." But Terriberry found no evidence that non-Catholic patients were discriminated against in their treatment and care. He recommended that the two chaplains, who seemed to be out of sync with the patients, be dismissed but that the sisters be allowed to stay. Terriberry agreed that employing religious sisters at a federally run hospital was "not right in principle," but said the advantages outweighed the disadvantages. Replacing the sisters "would be difficult, if not impossible," he said, because regular Public Health Service nurses were unlikely to come to the leprosarium for fear it would make it difficult for them to get a job anywhere else.

The Daughters of Charity were there to stay, but the patients had had their first real taste of collective power. If they made enough noise, flexed enough muscle, they might be able to get what they wanted. As soon as word got out that the Protestant chaplain, who was popular among the Protestant patients, had been dismissed, Early and more than a hundred others signed a petition asking that the chaplain and his wife be allowed to stay. "To take them away from us so ruthlessly, and, apparently without cause or reason, well nigh plunges us into hopelessness, from a spiritual standpoint," the patients wrote. But their appeal was to no avail. The decision was final.[21]

Investigator McMullen believed that the religious controversy was largely due to the patients having too much time on their hands. "The great majority of them have nothing to do but to idle their time away and brood over their misfortune which, in all probability, will last throughout their lifetime," he wrote to the surgeon general. "It is believed that all of these lepers suffer more or less mental disturbance. In all probability this mental unrest, together with enforced idleness, has been largely responsible for the religious disturbances which occur at Carville." He suggested that the patients be paid to do work around the facility to keep them occupied and also to help them support their families.[22]

Terriberry reached a slightly different conclusion. He believed that confining sick people against their wills, with little hope of release, made them more difficult to control. He noted that patients at Carville "never feel well. . . . They see about them constantly the terminal results of the disease, and look forward to the time when they will be blind and helpless." This feeling of futility, he said, made them vulnerable to a group of patients who used the religious controversy to increase their own influence and "who believe that by constant agitation along political lines they may get themselves in a position to dominate the affairs of this hospital."[23] He had no idea how right he was.

Chapter 9

Jail within a Jail

IF THERE WAS one thing the patients lacked beyond all else, it was hope. Living conditions had improved, but there was still no cure or effective treatment. Carville residents were constantly reminded that they were not only lifelong prisoners but social pariahs.

For one, nothing left the compound without first being fumigated or thoroughly disinfected. Patient mail was routinely sterilized in an oven, heated for one hour at 130 degrees—even though the process seemed to do little more than brown the edges of envelopes and remind the recipient that the sender was someone to be feared. Jewelry was placed in a sealed jar containing formaldehyde for several days and money was dipped in a solution of Lysol or 70 percent alcohol before it could leave the property.[1]

Patients were cut off from the world in multiple ways. They had no telephone to use to call family and friends. They were not allowed to vote, the result of a state law that disenfranchised residents of Louisiana institutions, including prisons, "insane" asylums, and the home for "lepers." For no logical reason, the patients had no voice in choosing the government that confined them. In some states, a diagnosis of leprosy was grounds for divorce. Even worse, patients often lost custody of their children.

Dr. Denney and the federal government tried to make life better for the residents, and in some ways they did. The medical officer made a good first impression when he arrived in 1921 and immediately tore down the much-despised fence that separated the men and the women. Patients of the opposite sex were finally allowed to interact, except in their rooms, without fear of punishment. Denney even organized the first dance—an awkward event, by one patient's account: "The men huddled timidly against the wall, staring across the dining hall at the row of bashful women while the band played to an empty dance floor. It was not until Dr. Denney took the hand of one of his feminine charges and led her to the floor and Mrs. Denney did the same with one of the men that patients dared act like human beings."[2]

Denney was one of the nation's foremost authorities on leprosy and believed strongly in the therapeutic value of exercise and keeping the patients busy. In his opinion, lethargy was almost as destructive as the germ. By 1924, the patients had movies twice a week, a band, baseball, tennis, and even a nine-hole golf course. A wooden tower had been built so they could see the river and catch a cool breeze on a hot summer day. A patient-run library held hundreds of books, newspapers, and magazines. There was a small school for the growing number of children and illiterate adults, although the teacher was one of the patients and attendance was not enforced.

Denney bragged in 1926 that they also had built a rudimentary lab, X-ray department, and surgical facility. Patients were given regular baths, massages, and ultraviolet-light treatments to relieve their nerve pains, numbness, and ulcers. They also received dental and eye care. A dairy at the rear of the property housed eighty cows to provide fresh milk for both the patients and the staff, which now included kitchen workers, groundskeepers, orderlies, and doctors.[3]

More than thirty single-story wooden cottages had also been constructed to serve as the patients' dorms. Each cottage had twelve private rooms, a small recreation area, and a screened-in porch where patients could sit without getting attacked by mosquitoes. The dorms were lined up like military barracks around a central courtyard and propped up on stilts to avoid the occasional floods, and patients were able to walk or bike for miles along the open-air corridors that connected them. A tea garden with a fountain had even been built in another courtyard next to a new mess hall. Denney said the goal was "to give each patient a room and surroundings which might be considered as his home."[4]

But a real home it was not. It turned out that Denney was also a believer in strict order and rules. Card games, which sometimes got rowdy, were not allowed past eight o'clock; lights had to be out by ten. He also drew up a list of regulations surprisingly similar to the dictates of Sister Benedicta. Patients were forbidden from leaving the grounds or coming in physical contact with anyone who was not a patient or member of the staff. Although he had removed the barrier between the male and female dorms, Denney forbade members of the opposite sex from communicating unless "authorized." What patients found most offensive was the language he used, calling his rules "Regulations for the Apprehension, Detention, Treatment, and Release of Lepers." Violators were warned that those found "guilty of an offense" faced suitable punishment, including "isolation and confinement." In the most serious cases, they would be "awarded imprisonment" with hard labor.[5]

The patients rightly complained that they were being treated like criminals rather than sick people stuck at the hospital through no fault of their own. Denney wrote that "to contract leprosy is not a crime. It is, in most cases, unavoidable." But he added, "Once a leper is in detention, however, it is a crime against society for him to abscond and subject his fellow human beings to the risk of contracting a malady that is practically incurable. To restrain such an individual is for the public good."[6]

Patients responded by running away. Confined to a lifetime of isolation, with faint hope of a cure, they had little to lose. Twenty-five patients absconded in 1926, and thirty-three fled the following year. Denney asked the surgeon general for more money to build a jail with up to thirty-two cells, where absconders could be punished. The Daughters of Charity had set aside a small building where runaways were confined for twenty days for a first offense, and twenty days more for each additional offense.[7] When the federal government took over, it increased the sentence to thirty days, and Denney said the three-room jail used for absconders and a similar structure for the "insane" were insufficient.

Denney complained that he had too many troublesome patients to handle, including an "insane Chinaman who has a somewhat unpleasant tendency to entertain himself by smashing chairs against walls and windows, and occasionally in the proximity of the heads of his fellow patients." This was likely the same "insane" Chinese man who had come from St. Louis with Hazel Deuser.[8] Denney reported that he also had in his care an "insane Spaniard" who had "fire-bug proclivities" and tried "to incinerate himself and one of the infirmary buildings."[9] There were other troublemakers, too, like Willard Centlivre, who was back at Carville after fleeing to Washington and falsely alerting authorities that the nation's "lepers" were preparing to invade. "The only way to keep this gentleman in detention, in my opinion, is to put him under lock and key where his friends will have no opportunity to encourage him into more bedevilment," Denney wrote to his bosses.[10]

The doctor was almost surely referring to the influence of John

Early, who remained the biggest thorn in the hospital administrator's side. A visiting psychiatrist who observed Early over a three-year period described him as "hostile and suspicious . . . restless and agitated." He said the patient exhibited "delusions of persecution" and "mental disturbance of a paranoid type not unlike the psychotic reaction of prisoners."[11] Incarcerating sick people was no easy task.

———

In 1928, John Early was stewing in the cinderblock building that now served as Carville's jail. It was not his first time behind bars at the hospital. Once—after escaping to Washington to protest how poorly the federal leprosarium was being run—he ended up being confined for thirteen months. His sentence kept getting extended because he refused to pay a $500 bond. He insisted that he did not have the money and that his hands were in no condition to do manual labor, his other option for getting released. Early told hospital administrators instead, "You will have to carry me out of your jail a corpse before I surrender to such an unjust, unfair sentence." Eventually, a face-saving solution was found. Early agreed to pay the government a nickel, after he noted that the regulations set no minimum amount for the bond. His offer was accepted and he was released from the jail.[12]

Now he was serving a six-month sentence for escaping again, this time to see his family in North Carolina. This latest escape was different. Hospital officials had decided in the spring of 1927 that Early was well enough to visit his aging father and they granted him a thirty-day leave. But North Carolina health authorities refused to let Early into the state. So he snuck out of Carville, hopped on a train, and made his own way to the family's home in the remote western mountains of North Carolina. He stayed outside in a tent to avoid contaminating the rest of his family.[13]

Early was able to elude authorities until August, when they got word that he was hiding on his brother's hilltop property outside the town of Tryon. A posse of federal and local law enforcement officials drove in a caravan up a narrow mountain road to reach the site but when they got there, Matt Early insisted that his brother was gone. A county sheriff decided to search the area anyway and discovered the fugitive patient crouched in the bushes, holding a Winchester rifle. The officer tried to persuade John Early to turn himself in, but he refused to budge. He shouted out that it made no sense for authorities to track him down in these remote mountains, where he was already isolated from the public, just so they could take him back to Carville to be isolated again. He argued that he should be left alone.

Soon, several of Early's relatives emerged from the house. They were all armed, men and women alike, with pistols in holsters strapped to their belts. They insisted that Early was causing no harm and they were willing to take care of him. But the authorities said the patient had to go back. For two hours, the standoff continued. Finally, Early relented, after he was promised that his brother could accompany him back to town. "He left calmly but with a trace of bitterness, only half assured that he will be given another opportunity to return to the mountain country he loves," wrote a reporter who had accompanied the lawmen.[14]

When Early returned to Carville, he was confined to the new one-story jail that had been constructed next to the patients' cottages. The jail was smaller than what Denney had wanted. It had twelve cells, centered around a small courtyard, with bars on the windows and doors. It was also surrounded by a chain-link fence topped in barbed wire, essentially a jail within a jail. Early complained that the twelve-by-twelve-foot cells were stifling hot in the summer and damp and cold in winter. "If I had not had the means to buy linoleum that I have put on the damp, cold concrete floor, I would have fared much worse with the cold, and without doubt, worse for the health of my old and weakened state of being," he wrote.[15]

The jail wasn't only for absconders. There were real criminals who also required confinement, which posed a special problem for hospital authorities. The same month that Early was returned to Carville, a patient named Edward Payton killed another patient, Lloyd Richardson, shooting him nine times with a gun that he had apparently smuggled in.[16] Payton claimed that Richardson was bullying him and he saw no other escape since they were stuck together at Carville for life. Payton was arrested and charged, and a trial was scheduled in Baton Rouge. On the appointed day, the courtroom was filled with curious spectators, although they stayed clear of the center aisle, where the defendant was expected to enter. Some in the overflow crowd peered in through the windows or watched from the balcony. "Silence fell over the assemblage as the door to the rear of the courtroom opened and the leper was ushered in, and there was not even a suppressed murmur as the spectators beheld the accused for the first time," reported the local newspaper. Payton was dressed in dark blue trousers and a white shirt, with a black bow tie and a green-and-black plaid sweater. He "appeared to cower and shrink from the gaze of the onlookers who watched him in silent horror and pity."

Outside in an ambulance, ten Carville patients sat waiting to be called in as witnesses. But Payton pleaded guilty to second-degree murder before their testimony was needed.[17] The judge sentenced the defendant to ten years in prison, but recognized that no prison wanted an inmate with leprosy. So the judge declared that Payton should serve his time in "whatever institution the attorney general of the United States shall designate," which, of course, turned out to be the Carville jail. Payton and the other ten patients returned to the hospital together.

The patients were upset by Payton's incarceration at Carville, but not nearly as much as they had been several years earlier. Patient George Beaurepaire had escaped to New Orleans, where he allegedly killed his wife on Bourbon Street with a gun (although some reports said he choked her) after she threatened to turn him in. He was indicted for murder, but then prosecutors had second thoughts. How could they put him on trial without jeopardizing public health? The U.S. surgeon general suggested confining Beaurepaire in the courtroom in a glass cage equipped with a megaphone. But the district attorney concluded that trying someone with leprosy was too great a risk and he dropped the case. Instead, he sent Beaurepaire back to Carville, reasoning that the accused murderer would be just as isolated there as he would be if he were sent to prison. But since Beaurepaire had not been convicted of a crime, he was free to roam the grounds like the other patients, who were extremely upset that they were treated the same as someone indicted for murder.[18]

Early's latest stint in the Carville jail only increased his bitterness about how leprosy patients were still viewed. He spent his long, lonely hours there writing a 235-page memoir, into which he poured twenty years of rage. Early complained that he had been hunted down like a wild animal even though he posed far less danger to the public than tens of thousands of people who walked around freely with syphilis and other highly contagious diseases. "The methods being used in dealing with these John Early Cases, in this age of science, modernity and non-superstition, are not one whit removed from the superstition of hanging witches and ducking scolds," he wrote. "Here they have him . . . in a dank concrete cell . . . locked up like a desperado . . . without trial or redress . . . refused the common privileges of a criminal—exercise and religious services . . . and forced to eat cold food . . . all in jeopardy of his health . . . mind and body . . . under the claim of 'protecting public health.' "[19]

Ironically, the Public Health Service declared shortly after Early was released from the jail that he had "recovered" from his disease and was free to leave Carville. Denney privately joked that they might have to "hog tie" Early and drag him out because the longtime patient appeared so confused when he was told he could leave. In fact, Early's symptoms frequently came and went, so it wasn't clear whether he had really recovered or the government was merely eager to get rid of him. The Public Health Service issued a news release in late 1928 calling Early's release "another triumph in modern medicine" and crediting his "cure" to chaulmoogra oil.[20] Early went back to live with his family in North Carolina, but became ill again in 1930 and returned, a weakened and dispirited man. It was time for the baton to be passed to a new crusader.

Chapter 10

———·•◦•·———

The Hole in the Fence

SIDNEY MAURICE LEVYSON arrived at Carville on a Sunday morning in early 1931, wearing a brown tweed suit, silk tie, camel-hair coat, and spats. He carried matching luggage with his initials stamped on the side in gold and clutched issues of his cherished *New Yorker* and *Theatre Arts* magazines. It gave the other patients the wrong first impression, that Levyson was some rich New Yorker. In reality, he was a young pharmacist from San Antonio, Texas, who was a little frightened, truth be told. But Levyson was a fastidious dresser and fancied himself a man of the world.

What he found at Carville shocked him. He saw many of the three hundred patients who now lived there consumed by a hopeless apathy. "The listlessness with which they went about their daily lives appalled me," he later wrote. "They followed the medical routine grudgingly, if at all. They were interested in food, enthusiastically and primarily. They were interested in sex and sometimes, I think, even in love. All their interests were superficial, day-to-day concerns, makeshift vehicles of escape from despair."[1] Levyson vowed to change that. He was thirty-one, filled with ambition and drive. He refused to believe that he might be stuck at Carville for the rest of his life and become one of the "living dead."

Levyson was born in Gonzales, Texas, part of a large, extended Jewish family.[2] As a teen, he worked in his father's pharmacy in the small town of Boerne, north of San Antonio, and remembered seeing a mysterious woman who periodically came into town to visit her doctor. When she stepped from her carriage, her face concealed by a heavy black veil, people would point and whisper. The rumor was that the woman had once been beautiful, an actress or an opera singer, but that her face had been ravaged by a horrible disease. He learned later, while preparing chaulmoogra oil for her at the pharmacy, that she had leprosy. He was astonished that such an ancient disease still existed.[3]

Levyson was a handsome young man, with a thick head of dark hair, who liked to dance and write and go to the theater. He hoped to become an actor or a journalist someday, but his father wanted him to go into the family business, and as a dutiful son, he did. He became a pharmacist and went to work at a San Antonio drugstore. One day a customer, a local dermatologist, came in and noticed an unusual red mark on the young man's wrist. He suggested that Levyson come see him in his office. The doctor conducted some tests and eventually gave him the bad news.

"The room started spinning on its axis and I closed my eyes to shut out the dizzy motion," Levyson recalled. There had to have been some mistake. How could he be doomed to the same fate as the woman behind the veil? But his physician, like Edmond Landry's, tried to soften the blow. He reassured his distraught patient that people seldom died from leprosy and that it was barely contagious. He told Levyson, who was twenty-one at the time and otherwise healthy, that he could continue working. "Most people have such mistaken ideas about leprosy," the doctor said. "Nobody is going to catch the disease from you in casual contacts at the store or at a party. And it's not a disabling disease in its early stages. It's not necessarily disfiguring either. And with luck, we can arrest it before it gets out of hand."[4]

Levyson and his doctor tried for several years to contain the disease, using chaulmoogra oil to treat the symptoms. The young man opened his own pharmacy and led an active social life. He performed in local theater productions and went to dances, although he was careful not to get romantically involved, knowing the secret his body held. Gradually, the germ spread, with more spots appearing on his face and his eyes becoming swollen and red. Eventually, the marks became too obvious to ignore and Levyson stopped going out. He sold his business at a loss in 1930, during the Great Depression, and headed to New York City for medical help.

Unfortunately, he picked the wrong doctor, one of the few in the city who was a stickler for the rules when it came to leprosy. He noticed that Levyson had an open lesion on his skin—the one symptom that required the doctor to report his case to New York health officials. He chastised the young Texan for coming to New York and told him he should immediately go to the national leprosarium in Carville. Levyson decided to get a second opinion, but the first doctor, on finding this out, was furious. He called the Madison Avenue hotel where Levyson was staying and told the management that their guest from Texas had leprosy. The hotel owner asked the young man to leave—but also to pay for his sheets, which would have to be burned. Levyson was then taken by ambulance to a hospital in Brooklyn for observation, with an escort of police on motorcycles. "As I was rushed across the Brooklyn Bridge, sirens screaming, I felt like a criminal being hurried to his doom," he later wrote.[5]

William Danner, general secretary of the American Mission to

Lepers and a strong advocate of the national leprosarium, visited Levyson in the hospital and convinced him to go to Carville. Danner assured him that he would be well cared for there. So Levyson, in his camel-hair coat, was locked in a train compartment with another leprosy patient for the long trip south. They were accompanied by a doctor who was not very encouraging, telling Levyson that leprosy "was a form of sin" that only God could cure.

The Texan received another shock shortly after he arrived at Carville. Sister Laura Stricker, the admitting nurse, suggested that he change his name to protect his relatives. He was extremely reluctant at first, being the only grandson on the Levyson side of his Jewish family, "with a commitment to save the name from extinction." He had already been stripped of his freedom—losing his name seemed like the final insult. But Sister Laura was insistent. "You have done nothing to be ashamed of but there are some stupid people in the world and you must protect your loved ones from their stupidity," she said. "Choose a name you will be proud of some day." With that, Sidney Levyson became Stanley Stein, patient Number 746.[6]

Stein immediately stood out from the other residents. Besides wearing fancy clothes, he tipped a fellow patient, as if he were a bellhop, when he showed him to his room. Stein was placed in one of the twelve-person cottages that enclosed a central courtyard where, he later learned, patients had been buried before the federal takeover. Now, a single stone monument, listing the patients' names and case numbers, marked the site of the old graveyard. "But their moldering bones still lay there to fertilize the magnolias—and to remind us of our own destiny," Stein later wrote.[7]

The Texan was taken aback by the filth he found in his assigned room—unchanged sheets on the bed, smears of dirt on the walls, trash on the floor. "The whole place stank," he observed. Other patients soon dropped by, purportedly to help him straighten up the place, but more likely to size him up. As in any community, there were cliques. Each cottage, like a fraternity or college dorm, had its own character, because patients chose their housemates whenever they could. "There was a Mexican house, a Chinese house, a Filipino house," and three houses set aside for blind patients, wrote Stein. House 42 was known "for being a den of roughnecks" and House 31 was home to the "lily-whites," or women of higher moral standards.[8]

Each new arrival at Carville was greeted with great interest and speculation. Would the newcomer fit in, and with whom? Joe Trahant, a Spanish-American war veteran—one of thirty-two, including Early and Koll, who would end up at Carville—was the first to welcome Stein, with a bottle of whiskey. Trahant told the Texan that he frequently escaped from Carville through the "hole in the fence." That was what patients called an opening in the chain-link barrier along the river road, just outside the view of the guards at the front gate. It wasn't so much a hole as a section of fence that had been pulled up from the ground just enough to crawl under. For decades, patients would sneak out, sometimes to party for the night, sometimes to leave forever. Even for those patients who never crawled through the "hole in the fence," it was a symbolic gateway to the outside world, a sign they could leave if they really wanted to.

Trahant told Stein that during his most recent escape, he had joined the Houston police force, something Trahant found especially amusing because he had once been a professional train robber. The next patient to drop by told Stein he was a Talmudic scholar from Philadelphia. He said there had been another Talmudic scholar at Carville but he killed himself by drinking Lysol after he learned that he was to be deported back to his native Russia. Stein was understandably unsettled. "Was that a hint, on my first night at the national leprosarium, of what might be in store for me?"[9]

What he found most disturbing, though, was the patients' apparent acceptance of their dismal fate. "They were a curious combination of rebel and submissive dependent. They resented being shut away against their will, yet they were complacent about being wards of the Government," said Stein.[10] Of course, this was the Great Depression, a time when many people living outside Carville were devastated by economic loss. Some of the patients were better off under government care than they might have been at home. They received free food, housing, and medical care, and were insulated from much of the nation's economic woes. It was no wonder they were a little complacent, although many of the patients were distressed knowing that their loved ones were suffering and there was little they could do to help. Edmond Landry told family members that he preferred not to read the newspapers or listen to the radio because it only made him worry about things over which he had no control.

Still, Stein found the hospital to be an intriguing place. Carville was an eclectic community, more diverse than anywhere he'd ever been. People from all walks of life had been thrown together in this tucked-away enclave, probably for life, rich and poor, young and old, male and female—although men outnumbered women two to one, for some unknown reason. Almost every ethnicity was represented. There were Asians, Hispanics, Caucasians, African Americans. About a third of the patients were immigrants, mostly from Mexico, where the disease was more common. At a time and place—1930s rural Louisiana—when many of the patients would never have crossed paths, Carville shoved them together. Housing was segregated at the time; whites and "coloreds" lived in separate dorms. They also ate at separate tables. But patients of every race worked, prayed, and played together. Blacks and whites were paid the same salary for doing the same work at Carville.[11] They also studied in an integrated classroom at a time when that was unheard of in much of the country.

Mycobacterium leprae did not discriminate. "Horizontally, Carville was a cross-section of the world's races and nationalities; vertically, it cut through all social and economic strata," observed Stein.[12] The patients were sharecroppers and wealthy businessmen and everything in between. Among those he met was a high-ranking naval officer who was a graduate of Annapolis and scion of a socially prominent family. Another patient was a former businessman who for years had represented a big U.S. importer in China. Another man's family was so poor, on the verge of starvation, that he was suspected of stealing funds from the patients' canteen to help them buy food. Some patients set up extensive gambling and bootlegging operations. Billy Lee, the political hack from New Orleans, grew marijuana. One of his buddies, Slim Gatt, commandeered a shower stall in one of the bathrooms, installed a fifty-gallon cask, and made wine that he bottled and sold.[13] Other patients put their entrepreneurial skills to work repairing bicycles, styling hair, cleaning clothes, and even running a Chinese lunch shop out of one of the cottages. A whole new community was starting to take shape, and for the most part Dr. Denney and the Daughters of Charity allowed it to happen, believing that a thriving, active social life would discourage people from running away.

Stein wanted to motivate the patients to do even more to take control of their lives, but he was pretty much on his own, with John Early now bedridden. The "obstreperous mountaineer," as Stein called him, was losing his eyesight, his energy, and, some suspected, his sanity after years of confinement. Stein was also relatively new to Carville and had yet to make a good impression on his fellow patients. He got his first chance to do so from Edmond Landry, who had been a patient for more than six years by the time

Stein arrived. Landry routinely used money collected by the What Cheer Club to provide entertainment for the patients and was in the midst of organizing a minstrel show when he became too ill to continue.[14] Stein, the amateur thespian, agreed to take over. He wrote to his mother in Texas and asked her to send his tuxedo and a book of vaudeville jokes. He ordered rhinestone jewelry for the female performers. They practiced their routines in a room above the X-ray lab, accompanied by an all-patient band called the Seven Hot Rocks. When the curtains were raised on the makeshift stage and the cast burst out with "'Sing, You Sinners!' the audience gasped and applauded wildly," Stein later recalled. "The show was an unqualified hit."[15] He had made his mark.

Stein also loved to write, and now that he could no longer be a pharmacist, he decided to give journalism a try. He suggested to fellow patient David Palmer that they start a newspaper. Palmer was a former marine who likely contracted leprosy as a child in India, where his parents had worked as missionaries. He was one of the thirteen patients who were brought down to Carville from Massachusetts's Penikese Island when the federal government took over, and he was still bitter ten years later about being confined. A newspaper, where patients could express their opinions and learn the latest gossip, seemed like a good idea. Stein asked Dr. Denney for permission, and much to his surprise, the medical officer gave the okay. The patients decided to name the weekly publication *The Sixty-Six Star* after the hospital's official designation, U.S. Marine Hospital Number 66.

The first issue came out on May 16, 1931, a little more than two months after Stein's arrival at Carville. Palmer was the editor in chief and Stein was the managing editor. They promoted the publication as "a Newspaper Devoted to the Interests of the Colony." "We hope that our modest efforts will meet with the approval of our fellow patients, and it is our ambition to issue a weekly sheet of breezy up-to-the-minute material," they promised. The first issue was two mimeographed sheets filled with patient gossip ("Mrs. Marie Moore enjoyed a visit from her daughter last Sunday," "Buddy celebrated his ninth birthday yesterday"), a sports column, the movie schedule (*Laughter*, starring Nancy Carroll and Fredric March), and the Sunday night dinner menu ("roast Louisiana capon with giblet dressing and cauliflower"). Subscriptions were one dollar a year, and before long almost all of the patients had subscribed, lured in part by the offer of a free fountain pen. It turned out, however, that the pens, which Stein had ordered in bulk through the mail, did not work.[16]

It didn't take long before the paper took on a hint of rebellion, with a feature called *The Adventures of Poor Egbert* about a fictitious newcomer to the hospital. The running comic strip poked fun at the hospital administration and the patients' unfortunate plight. As the story went, Egbert was assured by doctors when he arrived at Carville that he would be there for only two or three months and he naïvely believed them. All the other patients knew that he'd been duped. In one strip, a doctor told Egbert that if he followed the rules, "You won't be here long." The doctor then added as an aside: "You'll be in the graveyard."

The paper soon became a forum for patient grievances and got its first real taste of the power of the press when it covered complaints about the poor quality of Carville's movie projector. The sound didn't sync up with the picture and there was always a break in the show when the reels of film had to be changed halfway through. This was a big deal for the patients, who had little else to look forward to for entertainment. The issue drew a flurry of letters to the editor and eventually caught the attention of the assistant surgeon general, Frederick Smith, who received a copy of the paper in Washington. There wasn't enough money in Carville's budget to buy a new projector, but Smith was sympathetic. He arranged to have several carloads of beef and a load of hogs sent to Carville from another public health hospital to free up funds— which otherwise would have been spent on food—to buy a new projector. The news was so big that the *Star* rushed out a special edition to alert the patients. The staff wore old clothes and black-face ("Why, I shall never know," Stein later wrote) to distribute the paper in the cafeteria, shouting, "Extra, Extra."[17] Stein knew that, while the projector issue might be trivial to some, the paper's success was not.

The patients were slowly becoming energized, encouraged by people like Sister Catherine and some influential outsiders. In June of 1931, about two dozen patients, all veterans, stood along the low hedge that divided the property, waiting for a special group of visitors. The Louisiana commander of the American Legion, Sam Houston Jones, and several other legionnaires had agreed to come to the leprosarium to meet with the vets and to hear their complaints about how they were being treated. Jones, who would later become Louisiana's governor, was uneasy at first about meeting the leprosy patients. He had no idea what to expect. "They did not offer to shake hands. Their faces did not smile; it was as if they had forgotten how," he recalled. Another legionnaire eventually learned that the patients were afraid to shake hands because they feared that visitors would return home worried about contamination and never come back again.[18]

The legionnaires soon realized that the patients had a lot in common with millions of other veterans represented by the American Legion. "Mr. Jones, we're on the bottom," one patient told the commander as they sat together under a live oak tree. "You won't find anybody lower than we are." The patients said that they wanted better recreation facilities and more contact with the outside world and that Carville was in desperate need of a modern infirmary. Jones and his colleagues were supportive. They also saw an opportunity. The American Legion was in the middle of a bitter national campaign to secure more government help for veterans, especially better health care and benefits for those who had been disabled during World War I. The needs of the Carville veterans meshed perfectly with that campaign, and these patients were certain to elicit public sympathy. The men had fought for their country and contracted a terrible disease but were now treated like prisoners. They were even denied the right to vote. While the source of their leprosy could not be identified with any certainty, it was likely that most of them had picked up the disease while serving overseas, especially in the Philippines. "They were morbid, discouraged, inwardly sick," Jones later wrote. "Certainly, they had been neglected by the Government. Nearly all of the twenty-three were entitled to service-connection [compensation] for their disability; but they had received nothing."[19]

Jones had an idea. He advised the patients to form their own American Legion post at the leprosarium. "In union, there is strength," he told them. "You poor bastards here, twenty-three of you, are helpless. But with a million Legionnaires behind you . . ."[20] A few days later, on the Fourth of July, the Legion sent two of its local baseball teams to play an exhibition game at Carville, and that night they sent a band from Baton Rouge called the Ramblers to play for a patient dance. The Carville veterans soon formed their own American Legion post, and a new partnership was born.

In early 1932, top American Legion officials met at Carville with Dr. Denney and other Public Health Service officials to talk about the need for a new infirmary. They argued that the existing one—which was spread among several old patient cottages—was inadequate to handle the influx of patients. By now there were 340 and the hospital was still growing. Denney had been pushing for a bigger hospital for years but had been rebuffed by his superiors in Washington, who said there wasn't enough money in the budget. Now, with the powerful American Legion at his side, he was making headway. By the end of 1932, surveyors were staking out the site of a new, sixty-five-bed facility, which would also house an operating room, a modern laboratory, a pharmacy, an X-ray department, a dental clinic, and a morgue.

The patients suddenly felt they were having some influence over their own lives. Around this same time, Assistant Surgeon General Smith came to Carville and asked to meet with the staff of the new patient newspaper. He wanted to know what he could do to help. Stein mentioned that they had to rely on the mimeograph machine in the administration office to print the newspaper and that they could really use one of their own. Smith promised to get them one. It "was almost more recognition than we could bear," said Stein.[21]

The patient-editor decided it was time to start using *The Star* more aggressively. The paper was beginning to get some attention outside of Carville. Veterans' groups were subscribing, as were others interested in leprosy. Stein launched a campaign in the paper to address an issue that bothered many of the patients. They wanted to discourage use of the word *leper* and to have the illness referred to as Hansen's disease, so they would no longer be burdened with the biblical stigma. One of the paper's first targets was a national advertisement for a pain-relief product called Absorbine Junior, which used the slogan "Don't be a locker-room leper!" Stein published an open letter to the company that declared, "We do not spread obnoxious infections such as those afflicted with athlete's foot may do." He invited the company to send a representative to Carville to "learn something about us before you make such statements as are contained in your advertisements." There's no sign the company took Stein up on his offer, but this was the first of dozens of similar letters and editorials he wrote over the years, many of which would have a greater impact.[22]

The patients began to get more assertive in other ways, too, as though it had finally dawned on them that they had little to lose. They changed the name of the What Cheer Club to the more forceful-sounding Patients' Federation. They expressed outrage when a reporter with the *New Orleans States* newspaper wrote an article about Carville that described the leprosarium as a "veritable paradise," where patients were "happy and content" and would beg to be let back in if they ever ran away. The article was entitled "Looking In from Without," so *Star* editor Palmer wrote a scathing response, called "Looking Out from Within." He said that the hospital was "no paradise. Far from it," and that those who chose to return after leaving did so only because they were so despised outside they found they had little choice. Palmer said patients had great "bitterness against a society that, in order to protect itself against a menace which many of the more unprejudiced of modern scientists consider as hypothetical and imaginary as the giants and dragons of Cervantes, has robbed us of our liberty." He added, "Isn't it a wonder that we do not—like two cats tied together by their tails and thrown over a line—disembowel each other? That more of us do not go crazy? More take their own lives?"[23]

The patients used their newfound aggressiveness to push for a number of changes. In the spring of 1933, 160 patients signed a petition asking the Public Health Service to allow one of the residents, Louie Chee, to sell beer at a lunchroom he operated out of his cottage. Denney, who recognized that it was good for patient morale to have as normal a life as possible, gave his permission. Another petition requesting that beer be sold in the canteen was also approved.[24]

Later that year, an emboldened Stein wrote an editorial challenging the founding principle of Carville, that isolating patients would help eliminate leprosy. He argued that the policy was flawed and destined for failure because it discouraged people with the disease from coming forward for care.[25] "A modern colony ought to be a sanitarium for the patients to recuperate and regain their lost health instead of being a place for them to await death," wrote Stein.[26]

Then the paper went one step too far. In 1934, the *Star* got into a debate with the current Catholic chaplain at Carville over the significance of the "leper Mass" in Catholicism. The priest had written that the ceremony was "not intended to humiliate and crush the unfortunate, but to comfort and console him." The *Star*'s editors strongly disagreed. They called the Mass "about the cruelest practice that could ever be perpetuated in the name of religion." Among the authors of the editorials was the only black member of the newspaper's staff, Eugene Williams, a former dentist and a graduate of Dartmouth College. Stein considered Williams, who had been blinded by the disease and wore a tracheal tube to help him breathe, to be one of the most brilliant people he had ever met. Williams drew on his extensive knowledge of medieval history to counter the priest's arguments.[27] "We feel that the Church, both ancient and modern, has done more to keep the stigma of leprosy alive in the public mind than any other force," he wrote. "If the Church would be as energetic in trying to remove the stigma, which modern science has shown to be wholly unjustified, as it was active during the Dark Ages in instituting fear and horror, leprosy would be rid of the odium that now surrounds it."[28]

These were powerful words to use at a place where most of the patients were Catholic, and where the Daughters of Charity were the primary caregivers. It didn't help that Stein was one of the few Jews at the hospital. Other patients on the newspaper staff thought that he and Williams had crossed a line. In protest, they resigned or stopped showing up for work, and the *Star* folded. Stein was physically and emotionally beaten down. He was exhausted from launching the newspaper as the bacilli continued to attack his body. Stein had already lost sight in his left eye and some sensation in his hands. Now his right eye was starting to fail. It was time to take care of himself.

Chapter 11

Search for a Cure

DOCTORS WERE UNSURE what they could do for Stein other than keep him comfortable. They knew that the disease was caused by the *Mycobacterium leprae* bacillus, but they did not know why victims had such different reactions. It was a mystery why some patients became seriously disabled and others showed few symptoms at all. Or why some people seemed to miraculously get better and others did not. The patients were tested monthly for the presence of the bacillus but it was a very inexact method of tracking the progress of the disease. There was still a lot to learn.

A few years before the *Star* shut down, the Public Health Service had decided that it needed a lab technician to conduct more serious research. Sister Hilary, who was studying biochemistry at nearby Louisiana State University while she ran the Carville pharmacy, got the job and immediately went to work. Her new lab wasn't that much better than her original pharmacy. It was located in the patients' former kitchen pantry and the equipment was minimal—a few test tubes, a Bunsen burner, a poor-quality microscope, and some blank slides.[1] But Sister Hilary was used to making do with what she had and trained some of the patients to assist her. They learned to conduct basic lab tests so she could focus on studying the patients' blood chemistry and the impact of different treatments and potential cures.

It seemed as though just about every possible treatment and cure had been tried by then, including some farfetched ideas. When Carville was still the Louisiana Leper Home, a druggist from Key West, Florida, insisted that the bark from red mangrove trees would ease the patients' symptoms. He sent fifty pounds of the bark to the home to be used for both a lotion and internal medication, neither of which did any good. When rumors later spread that tea made from willow bark might help, enterprising patients stripped all the willow trees in the area and tried to sell the bark. Bags of unused willow bark were found in the attics of the old cottages when they were eventually torn down.[2]

When the federal government took over, the medical staff continued to test different treatments. They injected patients with smallpox virus and horse serum, tried fat-free diets, and experimented with ultraviolet-light therapy. At one point, Denney tried injecting patients with Trypan blue dye, which had little impact other than to leave patients with blue-tinted skin. The patients even conducted their own tests. After hearing reports that a Mexican doctor had seen promising results using something called Leprosal, the patients suggested that it be tried at Carville. When Denny refused, the patients had relatives from Mexico smuggle some in. They then enlisted a patient working in the clinic to administer the medication surreptitiously. It, too, did no good.[3]

Chaulmoogra oil was still the primary treatment for victims of leprosy, and a cure was nowhere in sight. Nineteen patients were "paroled" in 1929 with arrested cases, but thirteen others died and fifteen ran away, presumably frustrated that they weren't getting

better. Six patients who might have been paroled but had physical deformities decided to stay "rather than be subjected to the
hardships and humiliations, which are the inevitable outlook of
many paroled lepers," reported Denney. He claimed that optimism
at Carville was growing, but in reality the patients were increasingly pessimistic.[4]

Sister Hilary and her assistants were as eager as anyone to
turn things around. One of her helpers was former debutante
Betty Parker, who earned thirty dollars a month conducting routine urinalysis, blood counts, and tests for TB and syphilis. Hers
was one of the many jobs at the hospital that patients were offered
to earn some money and, as Denney said, "prevent morbid intro-
spection."[5] Sister Hilary tried to teach the patients who worked
with her about the disease that had engulfed their lives. The knowledge would prove especially useful later on when they started to
demand a bigger role in their own treatment. Parker was shocked
to learn how difficult it was to transmit Hansen's disease and that
it was far less contagious than tuberculosis. She was also surprised
that the bacilli that caused the two diseases were so similar that it
was sometimes difficult to distinguish one from the other. Under
Sister Hilary's guidance, Parker injected guinea pigs with patients'
blood samples to see if the animals developed TB. If they did, it
was a sign that the patient probably did not have leprosy.

Much of what happened in Sister Hilary's lab involved animals, such as rats, guinea pigs, monkeys, and sheep. Monday was
known as "gory day" because that was the day they collected blood
samples for a week's worth of tests and experiments. "There were
many inconveniences such as having to maneuver the sheep into
the laboratory and tie him to a post in order to bleed him for sero-
logical work," the sister said.[6] But try as they might, she and her
assistants were unable to duplicate the germ in the animals to be
used for research.

While she was conducting her lab work, Sister Hilary also began to experiment with photography. She set up a big flash-powder camera on the back porch of the cottage and practiced by taking pictures of the other sisters. One of her earliest photos shows an overexposed Sister Catherine, light bouncing off her white headpiece, as she patiently smiles at the camera. Sister Hilary hoped that with practice she could use photos to chronicle how the patients' conditions changed in response to alternative treatments. Again, her equipment was basic. She used the hospital morgue as a darkroom to develop the prints and to refine her technique. In 1929 alone, she ended up taking five hundred photos.[7]

————

New patients continued to arrive from around the country. Some came voluntarily, but others were brought there by force. One man from California showed up in chains and handcuffs. His wrists were so bloodied that no one could get the key to work in the lock and they had to cut the handcuffs off. It turned out that the man had been so frightened about where he was being taken that he jumped off the train in Arizona. After authorities apprehended him, they chained him behind a wagon and led him back to the train. The incident was so extraordinary that people at Carville talked about it for years.[8]

Most patients arrived more peacefully, resigned to their fate or convinced they were protecting their families by entering Carville. Amelie Landry came in 1934, at the age of twenty-seven, two years after her brother Edmond died. She had been ill for several years already and her move to Carville seemed inevitable. Twenty-four-year-old Johnny Harmon arrived in 1935, a year after his older brother, Elmo, was admitted. Elmo had shown signs of the disease since childhood, when his fingers were so numb he could stick a sharp needle through them without feeling a thing. Johnny was working as a draftsman at the Texas Highway Department when he realized he might soon be joining his brother. He noticed that the little finger on his left hand was numb. He also had an unusual blemish above his right knee. Johnny had visited Elmo at Carville the year before and was initially unnerved by the deformed faces and distorted limbs of some of the patients. But he was surprised to see that other patients looked normal. They also had a baseball field, tennis courts, a golf course, and plenty of food. Johnny thought that his brother "was happier there than he could ever again be at home," which eased his own fears about going to Carville.[9]

Johnny Harmon had hoped to put off the inevitable so he could enjoy his freedom a little longer, but he was given no choice. Right after he was diagnosed, an article appeared in the *Beaumont Enterprise* under the headline, "Health Officer Discovers Case of Leprosy in the Texas Highway Department," and his secret was out. When he entered Carville on August 2, 1935, Harmon discovered that conditions were even better than they had been the year before. The new infirmary had just been completed and the patients' wooden cottages were slated to be replaced soon with larger two-story dormitories. Social life had also become more active. Movies, dances, and parties kept the patients' minds off their problems, just as they did everywhere else in America during the Great Depression. Mardi Gras was by far the most significant and extravagant celebration in the state of Louisiana, and Carville patients—excluded from the rest of life—were not about to let themselves be excluded from that. They spent weeks creating costumes and building elaborate floats for a parade around the grounds that culminated in a carnival ball, complete with Mardi Gras king and queen. Harmon made a big splash his first year when he dressed up as Mae West, wearing a wig and a dress that his sister sent him from Texas.

Harmon was also among a group of patients who volunteered that year for the latest experimental treatment. Doctors were encouraged by the progress being made elsewhere fighting other infectious diseases, such as syphilis, yellow fever, and tuberculosis, and everyone at Carville wanted to add leprosy to the list. After years of disappointment, the patients were desperate for relief and became eager test subjects for almost anything that promised to ease their pain and speed their recovery. The newest craze was fever therapy. Doctors thought that intense heat might destroy the Hansen's bacilli. So Harmon and six other volunteers were taken to a hospital in New Orleans for days of testing. Harmon was asked to lie on a long tray, which was then inserted into a metal cylinder that resembled an iron lung machine. His head poked out one end as hot air was blown over the rest of his body and the temperature was gradually raised in an attempt to kill the germ. Instead, it almost killed Harmon. The treatment lasted four to six hours and by the fourth cycle, "I went hog-wild crazy and demanded that they let me out," he said. Harmon's temperature had been pushed up to 106.8 degrees.[10]

Another potential remedy had failed. When the exhausted patients returned to Carville, the Daughters of Charity noted in their annals, "Apparently this treatment is a disappointment, after the severe treatment that had to be endured."[11]

———————

In Jamaica, Queens, meanwhile, things were not going well for Morris Koll. He had spent the first few years after fleeing New Haven building a new meat business in New York and resettling his family. He had developed some ring-like marks on his face around 1924, but otherwise his condition was stable. His dermatologist even declared three years later that Koll was cured of leprosy, but that diagnosis turned out to be wrong. Red bumps soon appeared on his face and limbs, then spread to other parts of his body. Still, he continued to work. Business was good, despite the Depression, and he had a promising new venture—providing meat concessions for a chain of New York grocery stores. It was the latest trend in food marketing, and Koll was excited by the prospects for expanding his business.

But his health continued to deteriorate. Koll's eyes weakened as the bacilli attacked the surrounding nerves, inflaming his eyes and making it difficult for him to blink. Nodules on his skin grew thicker and his hands were beginning to curl into claws. He was also starting to rely on morphine to control the pain. His doctor tried to persuade Koll to go to Carville for treatment, but he refused. By 1934, Koll was completely blind and confined to the family's two-story house in Queens. He continued to conduct business over the phone, but handed much of the day-to-day management over to his eldest son, Leo. One night, Koll became delirious, probably from the morphine. He thought there was a lion in his room trying to turn his bed over. He tried to fight the creature off, but it turned out to be a woman the family had hired to help take care of him. "I hung on to her until I almost killed her," said Koll. It was time for him to go.[12]

Because Morris was blind, his teenage son Harold read the newspaper to him each day after school. On May 22, 1935, the lead story in the New York *Daily News* was about trouble brewing in Europe. The main headline read, "Give Us Our Colonies Back— Hitler." Harold likely told his father that the German führer was "thunderously cheered" by supporters as he demanded the return of colonies Germany had lost in the Great War. There was also a story in the paper about Congress trying to override President Franklin Delano Roosevelt's veto of a bill to give veterans more bonuses, the legislation that Sam Jones and the other legionnaires who visited Carville had been fighting for. Finally, there was a

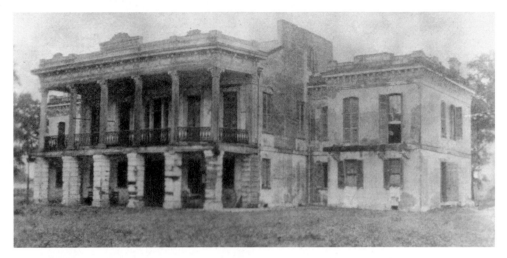

The Indian Camp plantation in Louisiana had been abandoned for years and was in ruins when the first leprosy patients were brought there in 1894.

From the collections of the National Hansen's Disease Museum, Carville, LA

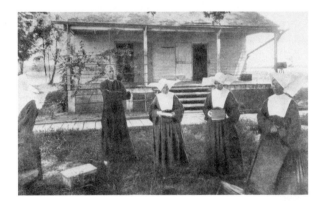

Four Daughters of Charity stand in 1896 with Father Michael Colton, the Leper Home's first chaplain, in front of one of the former slave cabins used to house patients. The sisters were recruited to serve as nurses and help rescue the failing home.

From the collections of the National Hansen's Disease Museum, Carville, LA

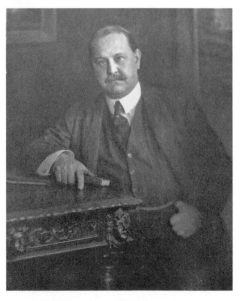

Dr. Isadore Dyer was a prominent New Orleans dermatologist who encouraged the state to establish a hospital for leprosy patients. He was the first president of the Louisiana Leper Home Board of Control, but quit in frustration because of lack of support from the legislature.

Isadore Dyer family collection, used with permission

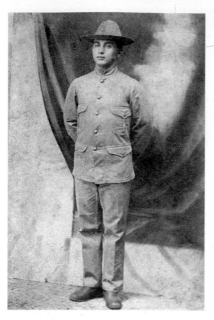

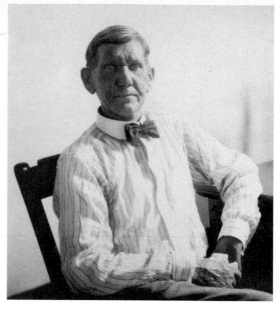

Morris Koll (then Kolnitzky) enlisted in the U.S. Army in 1901 at age sixteen and was sent to the Philippines to fight insurgents opposed to American rule. Koll likely picked up the germ that caused his leprosy while he was there.

Morris Koll family collection, used with permission

John Early, who called himself the nation's "most famous leper," confounded authorities with his disease. His plight led to creation of the national leprosarium in Carville, Louisiana, where he ended up as a long-time patient and agitator.

From the collections of the National Hansen's Disease Museum, Carville, LA

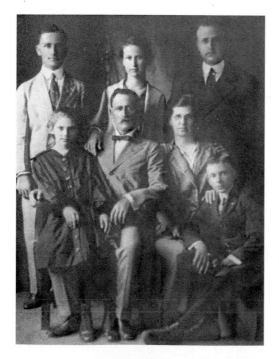

All five children in the Landry family of New Iberia, Louisiana, contracted leprosy and were sent to Carville, where they died across a fifty-eight-year period. A 1917 photo shows them in happier times. The three oldest children—Norbert, Marie, and Edmond—stand (from left to right) behind their seated parents, Terville and Lucie. The two youngest siblings—Amelie and Albert—are in front.

Landry Manes family collection, used with permission

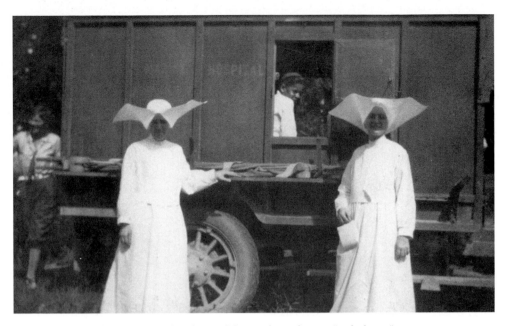

Two Daughters of Charity stand in front of the truck used as an "ambulance" to transport patients along miles of unpaved Louisiana roads to get to the remote leprosarium.

From the collections of the National Hansen's Disease Museum, Carville, LA

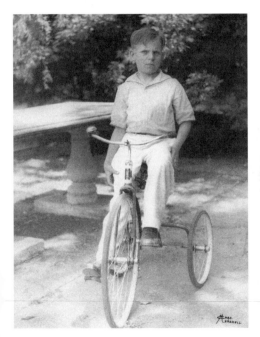

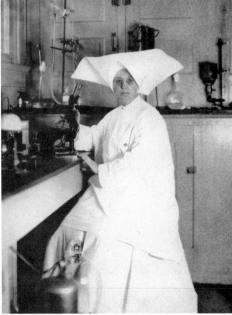

Seven-year-old Oscar Dempster was admitted as a patient around 1929. He lived at Carville until his death at age ninety-one.

From the collections of the National Hansen's Disease Museum, Carville, LA

Sister Hilary Ross became the chief biochemist at Carville and contributed to research that led to the discovery of a cure for leprosy.

From the collections of the National Hansen's Disease Museum, Carville, LA

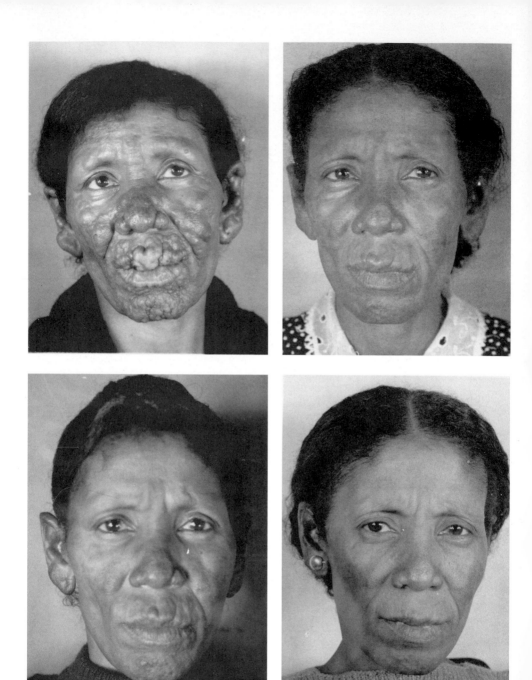

Photos of a patient taken by Sister Hilary illustrate the impact of a new antibiotic called promin, first tried at Carville in 1941. The first photo was taken in 1940 before treatment began, with the woman's face covered in lesions. Pictures taken in 1943, 1945 and 1947 show her dramatic improvement.

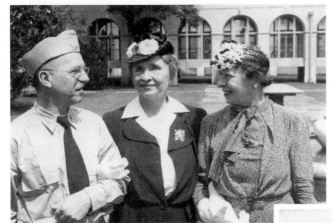

Medical Officer in Charge Guy Faget escorts Helen Keller (center) and her companion, Polly Thompson, during their visit to Carville in 1945. Dr. Faget was the first to experiment with using promin to treat leprosy.

From the collections of the National Hansen's Disease Museum, Carville, LA

The cover of the July 1945 issue of the patient newspaper, *The Star*, captured the patients' deep frustration at being confined against their will and unable to vote as the nation fought for freedom around the world.

National Hansen's Disease Museum, illustration by patient Johnny Harmon

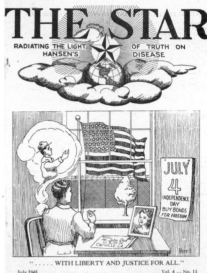

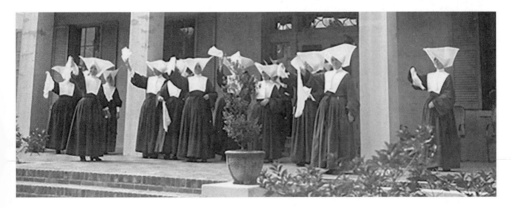

The Daughters of Charity waved their handkerchiefs to bid discharged patients farewell as they left the confines of Carville and headed to freedom. It was the opposite of the symbolic "burial" ceremony that patients endured in medieval times as they were cast from society.

From the collections of the National Hansen's Disease Museum, Carville, LA

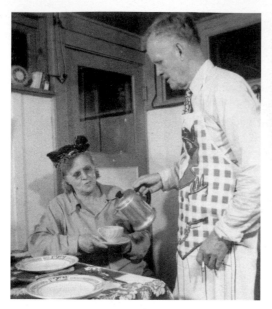

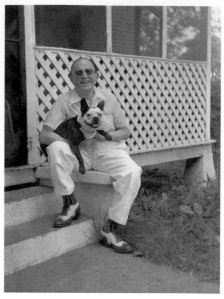

Hans Hornbostel serves his wife, Gertrude, tea at her cottage on the leprosarium grounds. The couple—both imprisoned by the Japanese in World War II—made a national splash when they revealed that she had leprosy and he wanted to go live with her at Carville.

From the collections of the National Hansen's Disease Museum, Carville, LA

Patient Stanley Stein sits with his dog, Bing, on the steps of his cottage at Carville. Stein was the editor of *The Star* and became an internationally known advocate for those with leprosy, which he fought to be renamed "Hansen's disease."

From the collections of the National Hansen's Disease Museum, Carville, LA

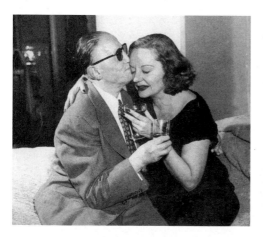

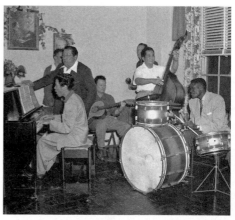

Stein was politically astute and enlisted outside support for the patients whenever he could. Actress Tallulah Bankhead became one of his strongest allies and invited Stein to New York for a whirlwind, highly publicized tour in 1951.

From the collections of the National Hansen's Disease Museum, Carville, LA

In the 1940s and '50s, life at Carville became more active as new drug treatments improved the patients' health. Music helped to keep their spirits up, and patients formed many bands, held recitals, and performed plays.

From the collections of the National Hansen's Disease Museum, Carville, LA

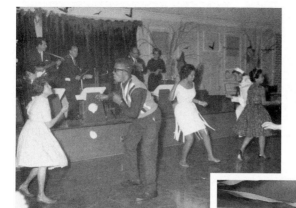

Patients enjoyed dances and sporting events with the help of neighboring communities. Outside bands often came to Carville to entertain. Public health officials believed that happier patients were less likely to resist their confinement.

From the collections of the National Hansen's Disease Museum, Carville, LA

Carville was an exceptionally diverse community, with white, black, Hispanic, and Asian patients mixing in ways unseen elsewhere in the country. Here, men share a holiday drink at the patient canteen in the late 1940s or early 1950s.

From the collections of the National Hansen's Disease Museum, Carville, LA

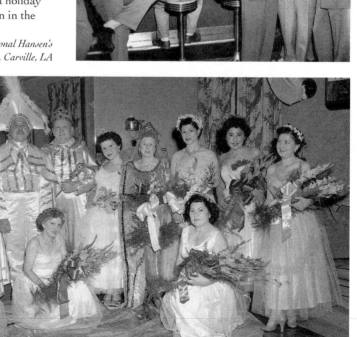

Mardi Gras was the biggest event of the year at Carville, as patients sought to have as normal a life as possible behind the barbed-wire fence. They spent months designing floats and costumes for the annual celebration and parade.

From the collections of the National Hansen's Disease Museum, Carville, LA

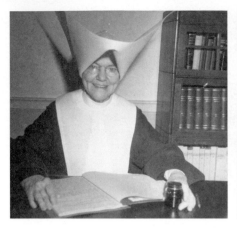

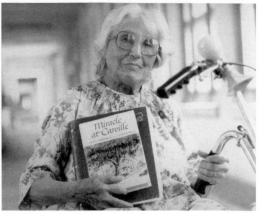

During her twenty years at Carville, Sister Catherine Sullivan became one of the patients' most outspoken advocates. She encouraged them to fight for their rights, often proclaiming that "mercy is no substitute for justice."

Courtesy, Daughters of Charity Province of St. Louise, St. Louis, MO

Betty Martin was a New Orleans debutante who came to Carville in 1928 and spent much of her life there. She wrote two best-selling books about her experiences and the great pain that she and others endured because of the stigma of leprosy.

From the collections of the National Hansen's Disease Museum, Carville, LA

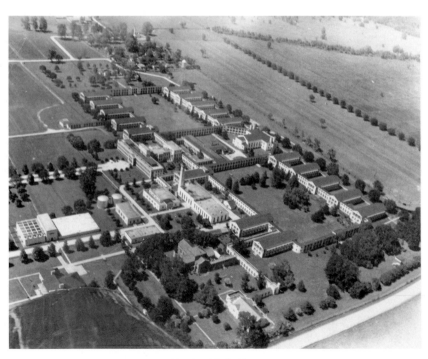

An aerial view of the Carville public health facility in the late 1940s.
From the collections of the National Hansen's Disease Museum, Carville, LA

reminder that it was only three weeks until a much-anticipated World Championship fight at Madison Square Garden between Max Baer and Jim Braddock.[13] These were likely among the last articles that Harold would ever read to his father. Later that week, the teen returned from school to find that his father was gone.

Two men, presumably health officials, had come during the day to take Morris to Carville along with three other leprosy patients from New York. If proper procedures were followed, the four patients were isolated in their own train car, under the watchful eyes of a health officer. Their meals were served using disposable paper plates, cups, and napkins. The utensils would later be soaked in carbonic acid to kill any germs left behind. Everything else the four patients touched in the train car on that long trip south—their bedding and curtains—would be fumigated with formaldehyde gas.[14] The patients were likely met at the New Orleans train station by the Carville "ambulance"—a box-like vehicle that seemed better suited for transporting livestock than people. The patients likely sat on wooden benches, unless they required a stretcher, which would have been placed on the floor as the ambulance bumped along miles of unpaved roads.

Koll, who was now completely blind, was likely startled by the near silence that greeted him as he was helped out of the ambulance at the leprosarium. The din of New York was replaced by birdcalls and the occasional sound of a voice echoing off the dormitory walls. Koll almost certainly felt his complete isolation from everything he had ever known. He was more than a thousand miles from home and, for him, at the end of the earth.

The Daughters of Charity noted the new patients' arrival in their diary that day—May 27, 1935. All four were immigrants. Koll was from Russia; the others were from Germany, China, and Greece. The sisters also noted that the Little Theater group, started by Stanley Stein, was scheduled to perform a show the following day in the canteen, a farce in three acts called *Second Childhood*. "This is the annual play; one of the big events among the patients," the sisters wrote.[15] But Koll would be unable to see, or even hear, the show. Like all new patients, he would be admitted to the infirmary for observation and treatment. He would eventually be moved to one of the dorms set aside for the blind patients.

It's not clear how willingly Morris Koll left his home, as ill as he was. In any event, he did not say goodbye to Harold, who would never see or speak to his father again. Harold's mother, Dora, swore all three children to secrecy about their father's disease and they dutifully complied. Leo took charge of the family business, but within a year he had lost most of their money by investing in a bad real estate deal. Morris knew something was wrong when the fifty-dollar monthly checks he received from his son to cover miscellaneous expenses at Carville suddenly stopped. "My son did not know how to handle the business; it was too much for the boy to manage, and the results are that we have lost everything," Koll told one of the doctors.[16] It was another burden for many of those who landed at Carville, worrying about how their families would survive.

Like the other patients, Koll lost more than his freedom. He also lost his right to vote, his name, and his dignity. He became Morris Krug, patient Number 1057. He was also constantly reminded of his outcast status. Koll was an avid Yankees fan and almost certainly one of the patients listening on the radio to the 1937 World Series game between the Yankees and the Giants. Sister Hilary recalled the patients' reaction when "the genial and jocular voice of the announcer said: 'Well, the umpire, you know, the umpire is the leper of the game. Everybody despises him but nobody touches him.' Oh, the pity of it!" she wrote. "Could you have seen the joy drain from their faces and the hard bitter looks as the radios were switched off."[17]

Koll did get to enjoy some of the recent improvements at Carville, including the new infirmary, which had a rooftop patio where patients could sit under an awning and enjoy a cool river breeze. He also witnessed an important change at Carville, a seemingly small development that made a huge difference in the patients' lives. One of their longtime complaints was that they had no access to a telephone to stay in touch with friends and family. The patients were so desperate at times that they would sneak through the hole in the fence and go to Baton Rouge, more than twenty miles away, just to place a call. Stanley Stein did that when he was worried about how the Depression was affecting his mother's finances. He paid a Carville kitchen worker twenty-five dollars—the amount Stein made in a month distributing chaulmoogra pills at the hospital—to meet him outside the fence and drive him to Baton Rouge so he could use a pay phone.[18] That all changed in 1936, when an American Legion official was visiting a patient who received a message from the front office that his mother was seriously ill and wanted to talk to her son. But the patient, a veteran, had no way to call her back. The legionnaire was shocked and immediately drove to Baton Rouge and appealed to the governor for help. A few days later a pay phone was installed on the wall in the patients' canteen. It was a party line that had to be shared with area families, but Stein said that for patients it was the most important event of the year.[19]

Around the time of Koll's arrival, the hospital was hit by a massive malaria outbreak. Nearly half of the patients, including Koll, contracted the disease, which weakened their immune systems. The outbreak led to renewed calls for the government to find a more suitable, less humid climate for treating leprosy victims. "Here we are situated in the midst of a malaria belt and at a level that is more or less menaced by floods," wrote Dr. Herman Hasseltine, who had recently replaced Denney as the medical officer in charge.[20] But his pleas did no good. The federal government had no interest in moving the leprosarium, which was no longer of much concern to anyone besides the patients, their families, and the staff. With the Depression and looming unrest in Europe, the nation had more pressing matters to worry about.

Within three years of the outbreak, 42 of the 155 malaria patients would be dead. Koll would be one of them. At the time of his death, he showed signs of advanced leprosy, with his forehead deeply furrowed and his face and ears marked by multiple lesions. Like many patients, he no longer had eyebrows or eyelashes and the cartilage in his nose had been absorbed into his body, as though it had collapsed. He had extensive ulcers on his arms, hands, legs, and feet and his fingers had stiffened into claws. The only personal property he still owned—an inner-spring mattress, a radio, and a small refrigerator—he left to a fellow patient. The other veterans at Carville arranged to have Koll buried in a small Jewish cemetery in Baton Rouge. In a letter to Dora, Dr. Hasseltine wrote that her husband "bore his lot with courage and fortitude." He was fifty-three years old.

That same year, 1938, John Early also died at the leprosarium he had helped to create. The nation's "most famous leper" was sixty-four years old. He had spent almost half of those years battling the stigma and ignorance that surrounded his disease, and trying to expose the absurdity of rules he and others were forced to follow. His most outrageous antics had long since been forgotten by the American public, but several newspapers noted his death. "For more than 30 years, Early's life had been a struggle not only against the disease itself, but against society," wrote one paper. "For more than three decades, Early was shunned by his fellow men as a thing unclean, and was hunted like a fugitive from justice." But in the end, Early saw "one of his dreams come true—Carville is now a government hospital."[21] At this point, though, it was unclear how much good it was doing.

Chapter 12

————— ·•·◆·•· —————

Until Leprosy Do Us Part

DEBUTANTE BETTY PARKER slowly adjusted to life behind Carville's barbed-wire fence. She made friends with the other female patients, played golf and tennis, taught at the school, and worked for Sister Hilary in the lab. She also followed the doctors' orders religiously, relying on chaulmoogra oil, warm baths, and ultraviolet-light treatments, in the hope that one or all of them might help her get better. Her case was extremely mild and she fully expected to be back home within a few months. The pink spots on her skin disappeared, but Betty was disappointed that she continued to test positive for the bacillus. Patients could be discharged only if they showed negative results twelve months in a row.

Betty was lucky in one respect. Shortly after she arrived, in 1928, a few relatively healthy patients from nearby states were allowed brief visits home, and she was one of them. Health officials were beginning to realize that if they eased up on some of the restrictions, even a little, the patients would be more content. Betty was able to return to New Orleans first in the summer and then to spend Christmas week with her family and her fiancé, Robert. He had visited her a few times at Carville, but he was also busy studying for his medical degree and his letters had become less frequent. During one of Betty's trips home, Robert admitted that he no longer loved her. She was upset but not completely surprised. It was common among the patients, whether married or not, to have those they loved decide that it was best to cut all ties.[1]

Maintaining relationships while confined at Carville was difficult, to say the least. Fighting a disabling disease and being ostracized by much of the world was hard enough. It was almost impossible to stay close to someone living outside. Family members could visit, but it was a difficult trip along unpaved roads. Phone calls were next to impossible and even letters involved the cumbersome and demeaning sterilization process. Sometimes it was just easier to leave the past behind.

But as the Daughters of Charity had discovered early on, the human libido is difficult to contain. The patients adjusted, especially if they were young and relatively healthy, and numerous relationships blossomed in the hidden enclaves of the 350-acre site, even among those with spouses at home. There was a saying at Carville that "absence makes the heart grow fonder, but not always for the one you left."[2] Many patients were drawn to each other by their shared despair; others simply longed for any physical contact.

Betty realized during her visits to New Orleans that, despite her family's deep love and their acceptance of her condition, she felt more at home with her fellow patients. No one else truly understood what she was going through. There was one person in particular who caught her attention. His name, an alias, was Harry Martin. He was strong and athletic, and as handsome as Betty was pretty. The two had much in common. They both arrived at Carville around the same time, under similar conditions. Harry was a nineteen-year-old student at Louisiana State University when he went to see a doctor about an irritating pink spot on his thigh. It was the same New Orleans dermatologist who had diagnosed Betty, and he gave Harry's father the same advice he had given to Betty's: Take your child to Carville immediately. Harry's father reluctantly agreed. He was worried about Harry's health but also nervous about the impact it would have on the rest of the family if word got out that his son had leprosy. The family even decided not to file a claim against Harry's $5,000 insurance policy—money they desperately needed—because it required revealing the truth about his medical condition. It was not worth the risk. The Martins (not their real name) sold their house and business in Mississippi and moved to New Orleans to be closer to Harry, and hopefully to avoid rumors about the whereabouts of their son.[3]

Though they were stuck at Carville, Harry and Betty did what young people do everywhere. They hung out together, looking for romance and fun. They joined other patients for impromptu dances on the wooden observation tower that had been erected so patients could watch the boats gliding along the Mississippi River. They performed together as the leads in one of Stanley Stein's first theater productions, a three-act comedy called *Stray Cats*. They celebrated Mardi Gras, with Betty dressed as a pirate and Harry as a country "hick." The young couple also strolled the grounds of the leprosarium on warm summer evenings, sharing their dreams about what they'd do if they ever got out. Betty had accepted by then that she might be staying awhile. "Sometimes we would stand still, sniffing the scent of automobile exhaust as a car sped past Carville and along the river road, and we would look at each other and sigh to be off and away," she recalled. "Starving people, it is said, dream of food, and in Carville we dreamed of motion, of getting on busses, trains, planes, anything that moves and goes anywhere."[4]

One day, Harry told Betty his real name, and she told him hers. It was the ultimate confidence that could be shared at Carville. They had fallen in love, although for Betty, a wedding was out of the question. As a devout Catholic, she believed that marriage meant children, and she did not want to risk spreading the disease or losing her child. Women who gave birth at Carville were forced to put their babies up for adoption, unless a family member agreed to care for the child. While the germ did not spread through childbirth, young children were believed to be more vulnerable to the disease and health officials were unwilling to put them at risk.

Even if Betty and Harry wanted to get married, they were not allowed to do so. Marriage between Carville patients was prohibited, although over the years many couples snuck through the hole in the fence and returned as husband and wife. They were usually split up when they got back, because male and female patients were required to live in separate dorms. Unless, that is, they were lucky enough to snag one of a dozen or so patient-built cottages located behind the dorms in an area known as Cottage Grove. It was one of the many oddities at Carville. After the federal government took over, some patients used scrap material that they found on the property—supplemented with supplies they bought from outside—to construct tiny homes where they could live with a bit of privacy and independence. John Early and the veterans were the first to build a private structure on the grounds, and others soon followed their example.

Surprisingly, the arrangement was sanctioned by the hospital's administrators. They believed that allowing the patients some freedom helped to boost their morale and made them more compliant about being confined. The cottages ranged in shape and size from little sheds to multiroom houses with running water, a kitchen, and a bath. Residents planted vegetable and flower gardens out front, and even had pets, which were not allowed in the dorms. The little houses were also the sites of countless dinner parties and card games. It was almost like the exclusive neighborhood in a tiny town.

Patients owned the cottages, which were sold or rented out when the owner was discharged, ran away, or died. The cottages were highly sought after, but a *Star* writer observed that "those who occupy them would gladly trade them for any mean hovel in the world—if only they could live there in health and without the terrible stigma which society imposes upon all who suffer from Hansen's Disease."[5]

Most of the cottage residents were couples, although Stanley Stein was able to rent one in 1934 with another male patient. That cottage had been owned by a former New Orleans socialite, who killed herself on the eve of her discharge rather than face the inevitable rejection of people back home.[6] Stein eventually purchased his own cottage for $500 and named it Wits' End. It became the site of many salon-like gatherings over the years.

Betty and Harry were more worried about their health than their future as a couple. Neither of them had many outward signs of the disease, but for several years their monthly tests continued to come back positive. Then, one month, Harry's test for the bacillus was negative, and it was the same the following month and the one after that. A discharge suddenly seemed within reach and the young couple was breathless. Twelve negative tests in a row meant freedom— or being "paroled" as "no longer a menace to public health," as the government's discharge papers so bluntly described it.

Then, a surprise. Betty got her first negative test, then another one the following month. By that time, Harry had had nine negative tests in a row, and they started to dream of the possibilities that awaited them outside Carville. Could they actually have a life together on their own? But when Harry's tenth test came back, it was positive, indicating continued presence of the bacillus. "We were so shocked we could not speak," said Betty. He was now stuck at Carville for at least another year, the earliest he could have twelve consecutive negative test results—a long shot at best.

Harry did what so many other frustrated patients had done

before him. He decided to run away. It was 1933, and he was in his mid-twenties and in relatively good shape. He did not think he would get any healthier staying at the hospital. If he wanted to have any life at all, this was the time to go. Harry asked Betty to leave with him, but she was torn. Betty was a follower of rules, and although she wanted to be with Harry, she worried about being apprehended by health authorities and bringing shame to her family. She also wondered what they would do for money if they escaped. Getting work was a challenge for anyone during the Depression. It would be much more difficult for someone who had no work experience and needed to explain a five-year gap in his life. Like many others at Carville, Betty wanted to abscond but was nervous about what kind of life she'd find outside the gates.

Surprisingly, Betty's parents made the decision for her. They told their daughter that she was wasting her life at Carville and should run away. It was a complete reversal from several years earlier when they were the ones who reluctantly took her to Carville and allowed her to be confined. Their daughter still had an awful disease, but from all appearances she looked perfectly healthy and, besides, her parents missed her. "Be ready to leave the night Harry leaves," her mother wrote. "Daddy will be with his [Harry's] father in the car."[7]

A few days later, after dark, the young couple ran across the golf course to the hole in the fence, Betty carrying a few of her belongings in a paper bag. They were accompanied by two friends who had come to see them off. The four patients crawled under the chain-link fence and hurried a short distance down the road so they would not be seen by the guards. They waited until they saw a car come slowly up the gravel road and its headlights blink three times. Harry and Betty said goodbye to their friends and rushed across the road. "In the car were both our fathers, and we knew what we were doing was right."[8]

Keeping the sexes apart—and avoiding unwanted pregnancies—was as difficult for the federal government as it was for the Daughters of Charity. The rule prohibiting patients from entering the room of someone of the opposite sex was routinely broken, or at least circumvented. When couples wanted to have a romantic dinner, they would set up a card table in the doorway of one of their rooms—with the woman on one side, the man on the other, and a candlelight dinner in between.

It was hardly a secret that many of the patients engaged in sex, if only to fill the long, lonely hours with someone who did not fear physical contact with someone who had leprosy. Assistant Surgeon General Terriberry reported in 1935 that while most women at Carville were "respectable and decent," a few appeared to have been professional prostitutes before they arrived. "It must be admitted, from all the evidence that could be gathered, that they are surreptitiously continuing their trade," he wrote. But Terriberry concluded that it would be nearly impossible to police such activity, given the size of the property and the patients' determination.[9]

A relationship was difficult to maintain with someone outside, not only because of the physical restrictions but because of misinformation and fear. As Edmond Landry learned, to his great distress, one's spouse could be extremely nervous about getting too close, despite strong evidence that the germ was not sexually transmitted. Landry argued with his wife that other patients' spouses often visited, and presumably had sex with them, with no ill effects. In his lengthy appeal to her in 1928, Landry told his wife that he thought his prayers had been answered when he met her, until "I found out that you would not have me for 'better or worse' but that you were with the rest of the prejudiced public and majority of wives who think that the unwritten law of marriage is 'until death or leprosy do us part.'" Like other married patients at Carville, he likely turned to another patient for intimacy out of sheer frustration. His letters certainly implied that he did. "Even though I am a 'leper' I am still human," he told his wife.[10]

Inevitably, some of those relationships produced babies, which made matters much more complicated. Perry Enriquez was a Filipino immigrant who worked as a lettuce picker in Salinas, California, when he was diagnosed with Hansen's disease and sent to Carville in 1936. Enriquez was in his late twenties, charming and handsome, with a thick head of dark hair parted down the middle. He liked to sing and play the guitar, and had an upbeat, optimistic view of life that even his illness could not contain. It was not surprising that a young patient named Maria, who arrived two years later, found Perry very attractive. After a few months together, they snuck off the grounds to be married by a justice of the peace. They returned to Carville but Maria was soon released after testing negative for the disease. Perry had to stay behind, but somehow the newlyweds continued to be intimate, because the next year Maria was pregnant. Perry ran away from Carville so he could accompany his wife to New York City, where their first daughter was born in 1940.

But Perry's health began to worsen and he returned to Carville later that year. Maria moved with their baby to White Castle, a small town across the Mississippi River, from which she could take a ferry to visit her husband. It was also easy for Perry to sneak out and visit her. Maria got pregnant again and a second daughter was born four years after the first. The couple wanted to give their daughters as normal a family life as they could, given the circumstances. Maria visited her husband regularly over the next nine years, with her two little girls in tow, sometimes dressed in pretty, ruffled dresses and white ankle socks, to see their father.

One photo shows the girls with their mother standing on the lawn near the Protestant chapel, flanked by two Daughters of Charity. After Perry was discharged in 1949, the family moved back to California where they could finally live together. His younger daughter, Dolores, recalled that she and her sister knew not to tell anyone about their father's disease for fear they might be forced to leave their new home.[11]

While children under sixteen were technically forbidden to visit patients, families often circumvented the rules by meeting at the chapel, something of a demilitarized zone near the front gate. Other times, one patient recalled, they would meet at the fence. "We had to kiss through the little holes," she said.[12] Another child remembered sneaking in to see her mother by hiding under a rug in the back seat of a car.[13]

The Daughters of Charity and other staff members usually knew what was going on but turned a blind eye unless they thought someone's health was at risk. It was the same old paradox for those living with Hansen's disease—they were considered a mortal threat one day, and relatively benign the next.

Johnny Harmon, the Texan who followed his brother Elmo to Carville, also fell in love. He was released in 1938 after he tested negative for the disease but was readmitted four years later when it reemerged.[14] A girl named Anne Triche had been one of his students at the Carville school during his first stay and she was still there when he returned. He liked her as a student, but she was only fourteen years old at the time. Now she was a young woman. Anne and Johnny got married in 1948. Since they were not allowed to do so at Carville, they arranged to meet at a church in New Orleans while both of them were on leave. When they returned, Johnny surreptitiously stayed in Anne's room when he could, but they eventually got their own place in Cottage Grove.

The Harmons did not plan to have children, especially because Anne's family was highly susceptible to the disease. The family home, located in a nearby parish, had even been burned down by local authorities for fear that the germs might spread. Several of her relatives were patients at Carville, including her mother and three of her brothers. The youngest, a sweet boy named Andre, was admitted at the age of four and was known as the "pet of the colony." Andre died of kidney failure when he was eleven years old.[15] Nevertheless, Anne became pregnant two years after she and Johnny were married, and they had to find someone to care for the baby or else it would be put up for adoption. Johnny tried to recruit his sister in Texas, but she refused. They eventually found a couple in nearby Vacherie—Anne's brother's in-laws—who agreed to take their baby son. In 1952, Anne got pregnant again. Fortunately, the Vacherie couple agreed to raise their daughter as well. It was a convenient, if unusual, arrangement, and the couple brought the Harmon children to see their parents as often as they could. Johnny and Anne would sneak through the hole in the fence and meet them two or three times a month on the levee. "We would have a picnic under the willow trees on the bank of the Mississippi River," Johnny recalled.[16] It was the only way they could see their children and watch them grow.

Other patients were less fortunate than the Harmons. Most of those who were parents had had to leave their young children behind in the care of spouses or other family members and, like Edmond Landry, seldom saw them again. Or, like Morris Koll, never did. One twenty-six-year-old Texas woman left six children, all under the age of ten, to come to Carville, where she stayed for the rest of her life.[17] Her adult daughters came to visit many years later but kept their mother's illness a secret.

The pain of separation from family was by far the worst part of being at Carville. To the patients, nothing else compared. Not the disease itself, or the physical confinement, or the loss of identity and rights. A March 13, 1940, entry in the Daughters of Charity annals was heartbreaking, but not all that unusual. "Poor Bobbie (a patient) weeps to-day over a letter received from the eldest of her three girls (her very own) saying 'It will be better, Mother, for you to give us up and don't write any more; just found out that they have it on my record at school that my mother is a 'Leper' in the Lepers Home. I intend to go to College and I don't want this record to follow me so hereafter will say that you are dead, and don't write any more.' Poor, heart-broken mother!"[18] A few years later, the sisters noted the return of a patient from Mexico: "He had eight children, none of whom he said wanted him and his wife had deserted him, so he had to come back."[19]

The pain wrapped itself around entire families, with children the frequent victims. Marie Guerre was thirteen years old in 1940 when both she and her older sister were brought to Carville. She was shocked to discover that their grandmother was also a patient there. Marie's father cried when he left off his two girls, but he worked on a tugboat that regularly went up and down the Mississippi and told Marie he would blow the horn three times when he passed to let her know he was thinking of her. "Being 13, I didn't want to miss it," said Marie. So she stood outside every day by the fence waiting for the whistle. "It came once out of the whole year. One time," she recalled. Marie thought her father no longer loved her. But a couple of years later, when after ten clean monthly tests she failed her eleventh—dooming her to another year of confinement—her father and his boss came to Carville, picked her up from her bed, and took her home.[20]

Things were especially difficult when patients got pregnant at Carville and did not have outside support as the Harmons did. The mothers were usually taken to a New Orleans hospital to deliver the babies, although the patients joked that most Carville babies were born on the way there as the ambulance bounced along the unpaved road. Some mothers didn't make it even that far. One night, several patients heard what sounded like a cat crying in one of the dorm rooms. When they opened the door, they found a female patient in a rocking chair cradling a newborn. Her boyfriend had just delivered the baby. When the doctor arrived, some of the other patients told him the boyfriend should be put in the Carville jail. "Heck no, he did a damn good job," the doctor responded. A Daughter of Charity nurse soon arrived and took the baby from the mother, so the child could be placed in the care of a relative.[21]

Other cases were more tragic. One female patient, who was already married but lonely without her husband at Carville, had a relationship with another patient and became pregnant with twins. The woman was distraught about having to reveal the pregnancy to her husband, but she had little choice so she went through with it. Both babies died shortly after birth, and the mother died soon after that, although it's unclear how.[22] Another female patient, who had to leave her four young children with their alcoholic father when she came to Carville, became pregnant at the hospital. Her baby was put up for adoption and died eighteen months later of unknown causes.[23]

Dr. Hasseltine, the chief medical officer in the late 1930s, tried desperately to enforce the no-fraternization rules in the dorm rooms. He even suggested at one point that female patients be sterilized before they married other patients, to avoid any "difficulties," although the proposal was dropped and might have had the opposite effect.[24] Stein said patients ended up calling Hasseltine "grandpappy" because more babies seemed to be born during his five-year tenure than ever before.[25]

Being in love was not much easier outside Carville for Betty Parker and Harry Martin. Betty was exhilarated at first to be home again after their nighttime escape, and to walk the streets of her beloved New Orleans. She had a lot of pent-up socializing to do and tried to resume her old life under her real name, Edwina Parra. She joined Harry and his family for a two-week vacation on the Gulf Coast and went to the Chicago World's Fair with a relative. She eventually got a job as a stenographer and Harry returned to college. Their new life together appeared to be going well, but they both knew they were living a lie. "The fear of stigma kept us in a prison," she later wrote. Betty would panic each time she ran into someone who might have seen her at Carville—a former patient, a worker, or a visitor—and could reveal her secret. She also constantly worried about spreading germs, especially to her baby nephew. She made excuses to stop him from climbing on her lap but was so sad about it that she would go into the bathroom afterward and cry. Betty and Harry were constantly on guard.[26]

Then Harry's health began to deteriorate. His vision was fading and one of his ears became swollen. Betty realized that the disease was overtaking his body. She had been reluctant to marry Harry before but changed her mind. She loved Harry and wanted to be able to nurse him if he got any sicker. Her parents made the decision easier by promising to care for any children they might have. The young couple got married in 1938, in a small, private ceremony, and tried to build a life together. But a year later, Harry decided he had to return to Carville. The bumps on his ear were becoming noticeable to customers at the small hardware store that he ran and his eyesight was getting worse. He was also worn down trying to both fight the disease and maintain the deception. Betty insisted on returning to Carville with him, even though she had remained healthy. It was where they belonged. "It offered now sanctuary," Betty wrote. "Outside, with health and vision changing, Harry was less free than he would be in Carville. Only there, among our own, could we let down our barriers." But she did not return with the same naïve optimism of twelve years earlier. "This time we would know that Carville was the end of the road."[27]

The Martins still felt compelled to conceal the truth. They told their New Orleans friends and relatives that they were moving to Virginia so Harry could get a new job.

The Carville they returned to was not the one they'd left five years before. There was a new Catholic chapel and the modern infirmary. Doctors had been hired to do reconstructive surgery on patients' hands and feet, and physical therapists helped the patients adjust to their disabilities. New fireproof dormitories and a huge recreation center were in the works. Still, some things remained the same. Betty and Harry were once again confined behind a chain-link fence topped with barbed wire. They once again lost their right to vote, and letters home were sterilized. They assumed their old aliases but were assigned new patient numbers. Betty, who had been Number 543, was now Number 1293. They also were not allowed to live together as husband and wife. After being greeted warmly by old friends and hospital staff, the Martins were put behind bars for thirty days, as punishment for having escaped.[28] Betty was isolated in a cottage with barred windows, while Harry was sent to the Carville jail. Afterward, they went to live in separate dorms. As Stanley Stein said, "Carville was still a pretty dismal place in which to spend the rest of one's life."[29]

Chapter 13

The Miracle

THE MARTINS WERE distressed on their return to Carville to see how many of their old friends were now in wheelchairs or had gone blind. All of the children they had known five years earlier were either dead or in advanced stages of the disease. "Each morning when Harry and I met in hydrotherapy one of us would ask in shocked tones, 'Have you seen so-and-so?'"[1] The 1935 malaria outbreak had taken its toll, not only killing many patients but weakening the defenses of others. Pneumonia and influenza hit the Carville community especially hard during that winter of 1940. Despite some improvements at Carville, doctors were still frustrated in their effort to find a more effective treatment or a cure for Hansen's disease.

Dr. Guy Faget, who arrived that summer to replace Hasseltine as the medical officer in charge, did not look like the person who would turn things around. He was a small, nondescript man with rimless glasses and a tuft of a mustache. He had gotten his degree from Tulane's medical school when Isadore Dyer was still dean

and then gone on to work at various Public Health Service hospitals over the next two decades. Faget's expertise was in tuberculosis research, not Hansen's disease, so there was no reason to expect
that he would make any breakthroughs in a field that had proved
challenging for so many others. He also did not make a good first
impression on the patients, with his crisp, bureaucratic style. Faget
seemed like someone who would be more worried about rules and
procedures than the opinions of incarcerated patients. He had the
"poise of a bantam rooster," Stein wrote dismissively.[2]

Stein was especially discouraged at this point in his life. He
had gone through an extremely difficult period following the shut-
down of *The Sixty-Six Star*. As his eyesight slowly disappeared, he
was tortured by extraordinary pain. His eyes felt as though they
were being stabbed with burning needles whenever they were hit
by bright lights. His hands had become increasingly stiff and crippled, and his legs were covered in sores. Stein finally checked himself into the infirmary in late 1936 and fell into a deep depression.
"My vision was failing, but I could see clearly what lay ahead for
me," he wrote.[3] By the end of the following year he was completely
blind. For a man who loved to read, Hansen's disease proved to be
doubly cruel. Not only could he no longer see, but his numbed fingers made Braille useless. He was now dependent on others to read
to him. The man who had invigorated the patients to act on their
own behalf was now paralyzed with loneliness and grief.

Sister Catherine came to the rescue. She had recently been
transferred to the Daughters of Charity motherhouse outside St.
Louis, Missouri, but remained a staunch advocate for the Carville patients. Stein was one of her favorites. The Irish Catholic
sister and the Jewish activist had much in common. They shared
the same sense of injustice and a strong belief that if the patients
did not fight for themselves, no one else was likely to do so. Sister
Catherine's favorite saying—"Mercy is no substitute for justice"—

had endeared her to the rebel Stein. On a visit back to Carville, she stopped by the infirmary to try to boost his sagging spirits. She suggested that Stein seek help from his family's rabbi back in San Antonio, even though it meant revealing the truth about his disease. Stein's mother had told friends and relatives that her son had to leave town because of a nervous breakdown, which for her, as for so many other patients' families, was preferable to admitting that someone they loved had leprosy.

Stein agreed to have Sister Catherine write a letter to Rabbi Ephraim Frisch, a copy of which Stein kept and cherished for the rest of his life. "Because I am a Texan," her letter began, "Carville has always appeared as another Alamo to me, where brave men and women . . . fight overwhelming odds . . . on a three-fold front: first, against a pitiless disease; second, they fight the age-old accumulation of ignorance, prejudice and fear; third, they must fight the bitterness and despair engendered in their hearts." Sister Catherine told the rabbi that "Sidney is one of the bravest combatants. You will extend to him, I know, the aid and encouragement of a friend."[4] Rabbi Frisch immediately responded with his support and eventually came to visit. Stein was comforted knowing that at least one person back home, besides his mother, knew what had really become of Sidney Levyson. It was a tiny sliver of recognition that the man he had once been was still alive. As Sister Catherine well knew, leprosy was more than a medical disease. It corroded the spirit of those who believed they had lost their identity and place in the world. Stein slowly began to recover.

By the time the Martins returned to Carville, Stein had rejoined the land of the living and was trying to figure out how he could once more agitate for better conditions. He and a small group of friends had discussed relaunching the *Star* but decided they did not have enough energy. That's where things stood in 1941 when Stein and Harry Martin helped to organize the dedication ceremony, complete with a dance and floor show, for the new patient recreation center, set to open in August. The dedication was an eagerly anticipated event, because the center was replacing an old wooden building that had served as the patients' recreation hall for years. The new one far exceeded their expectations. It was an elegant, spacious structure that reflected the design of the plantation mansion, complete with Corinthian columns, tall windows, and a second-floor balcony edged in cast-iron grillwork. The first floor held a modern theater with cushioned seats, a patient canteen, a post office, library, a game room, and meeting rooms. The second floor was dominated by a massive ballroom, perfect for Mardi Gras dances and Christmas celebrations. The hall was the product of a lobbying campaign by the American Legion and one of the clearest signs yet that the government was taking the patients' demands and well-being more seriously.

Louisiana governor Sam Jones, the legionnaire who had encouraged Carville's veterans a decade earlier to fight for better treatment, came that day to dedicate the building and uttered words that further inspired the already exhilarated patients. "Every great thing starts out as a dream for someone, and this recreation building has long been the dream of the American Legion and the patients of Carville," Jones told the gathering. Stein and his colleagues decided right then that they would restart the *Star* and use it as a tool to achieve some of their other dreams. The new paper would be a lot like the old one, but without *Sixty-Six* in its name. It would also have a new slogan that would run across its masthead for decades to come: "Radiating the Light of Truth on Hansen's Disease." There would be no question this time what its mission would be.[5]

The first subscriber to the reborn *Star* was none other than Guy Faget, the new medical director. In fact, he ordered two subscriptions. Faget was slowly endearing himself to the patients and

showed sympathy for their cause. In December 1941, as the Japanese attack on Pearl Harbor drew the United States into war,
Faget wrote a column for the reborn *Star* called "Courage." Sounding a lot like a military officer trying to motivate his troops, he
told the patients that they needed to take a more active role in
fighting their disease, that finding a cure required them all to work
together. "Knowledge and Experience are the generals of the defensive forces," he wrote. "In all chronic disease, such as tuberculosis,
diabetes, and leprosy, the patient's intelligence and insight into his
malady, as well as his cooperation with his physician, are of the
greatest assistance to his success." Faget encouraged the patients
to fight the "false propaganda" about leprosy. It was not a dread or
hopeless disease. It could be conquered. He also said they should
not be discouraged by the many failed medical experiments over the
years, because each one taught researchers something new about
the disease. "Therefore let us all cooperate and pull together—the
patients and the personnel. Together we will succeed; divided we
will fail."[6] He later echoed that theme in a speech honoring patients
buried in the Carville cemetery: "What does it matter that their
enemies were germs instead of Germans? . . . Each who died left
behind some bit of knowledge to fortify using [in] the future fight.
Let us make sure that they have not died in vain."[7]

These were powerful and inspiring words for those who felt
as if they were often treated more like numbers than people. But
Faget realized that he needed the patients' cooperation if medical
testing was to succeed. Science was on the cusp of many major
breakthroughs, especially when it came to fighting germs, and
Faget wanted Carville to be included.

Research was booming everywhere as nations headed into
the Second World War. Vaccines, antibiotics, and other treatments were being developed to conquer some of the world's most
dangerous diseases. The same year that the Carville recreation

center opened, scientists at Oxford University successfully used penicillin to treat bacterial infections. Two years later an antibiotic was developed to control tuberculosis. Other scientists were working furiously to find a vaccine that would protect American troops from illnesses such as influenza. Some 44,000 members of the U.S. military had died in the flu pandemic of 1918, and no one wanted something like that to happen again. Unfortunately, with war looming, discovering a cure for Hansen's disease was a low priority. But the patients were as eager as ever to get better. They closely followed the latest medical developments and prodded their doctors to be aggressive with experimental treatments.

In 1940, Carville's physicians decided to try injecting diphtheria toxoid into patient volunteers. They speculated that it might spur the development of antitoxins that would attack the Hansen's bacilli. An outside doctor, who claimed that he had success using the treatment overseas, visited Carville one day with before-and-after photos that seemed to show noticeable improvements in his patients' conditions. The Carville patients wanted to give it a try, although the doctors and Daughters of Charity were skeptical. The sisters wrote in their diary on March 19 that the new diphtheria toxoid treatment was starting that day, adding, "St. Joseph pray for us!"[8]

Initially, a few dozen patients were tested, but soon others were demanding that they be included as well. The doctors were reluctant, but eventually 230 patients, about two-thirds of the total population, were getting the treatment.[9] In the end, they were all disappointed. The injections did not work. Sister Hilary wrote that instead, "the majority of the patients under treatment got worse."[10]

It was not surprising, then, that Faget's next experiment attracted little enthusiasm at first. He had been following the latest tuberculosis research, his area of expertise, and noticed that physicians at the Mayo Clinic in Rochester, Minnesota, were getting some positive results using a new antibiotic called promin on TB-infected guinea pigs. Faget knew that the tuberculosis and Hansen's disease bacilli were similar and wondered what impact the drug might have on leprosy patients. He wrote to the head of clinical investigation at the Parke-Davis pharmaceutical company, the maker of promin, for more information and learned that another doctor had been testing the drug on rats with a disease similar to human leprosy. Promin had reduced the size of the rats' leprous nodules and increased the animals' survival time. The company offered to send Faget a free supply of the medication so that he could conduct his own tests on humans. Faget consulted with the other doctors at Carville, who had some reservations about putting the patients through more experiments after the disappointment of the diphtheria toxoid injections. But they finally decided it was worth a try.[11]

On March 10, 1941—when the big news outside Carville was the arrival of a new president at nearby Louisiana State University—six volunteer patients went to the infirmary to get their first injections of promin. The initial results were not encouraging at all. After several weeks, some of the volunteers developed serious side effects, such as anemia, allergic dermatitis, and nausea. Others complained that the daily injections were too painful. Dr. Faget tried different dosages and experimented with other ways of administering the drug to reduce the negative reactions. Sister Hilary spent long hours in the lab, testing the patients' urine and blood samples to determine how the drug was affecting their bodies so the doctors would know what adjustments needed to be made. She also photographed the patients to keep track of any changes in their physical appearance.

Many of the original volunteers grew discouraged and new ones were difficult to find. But a popular young doctor at Carville, Raymond Pogge, eventually came up with a more palatable version of the medicine by mixing it with glucose, calcium, vitamin B, and penicillin. The patients called it the Pogge Cure-All Cocktail and it became such a hit that volunteers began to sign up again for the tests. Slowly, patients taking the drug began to see changes. Leprous nodules and blemishes on several volunteers started to disappear after six months. Mouth lesions began to heal and breathing became easier for those with respiratory problems. The patients still tested positive for the disease, but the medication was having a noticeable effect.

Among the patients to receive the experimental treatment was Harry Martin. His legs had recently grown swollen and ulcerated. His arms and one of his feet were covered in ugly purple spots and his white blood-cell count was dangerously low. The new treatment seemed like another false hope, but he and Betty were desperate. They believed that Harry was losing his battle with the disease. Nothing else was working and the germs were clearly taking over his body. They reluctantly decided to give promin a try.

At first, the daily injections seemed to have little impact. Betty tried to keep herself busy working on *The Star* and practicing with the choir for a Christmas performance. After two months, Harry's condition grew worse. Betty stayed by his bedside on New Year's Eve as his temperature soared to 104 degrees and his face became swollen and red. The swelling became so bad at one point that he was almost unrecognizable. The doctors decided to stop the promin injections and gave Harry other medication to reduce the swelling. Within days, it was gone.

Then something odd happened. The ulcers on Harry's legs suddenly began to disappear. Within a week, he was out of bed and walking. Harry was getting better. "When the flare-up had completely subsided we saw the hideous ulcers that had existed so long were healing," Betty recalled. "We knew then. This was our miracle."[12]

The patients might have believed they had seen a miracle, but the doctors at Carville were far more cautious. They were not ready to declare victory. As with many scientific discoveries, the significance of this one was not immediately apparent. Dr. Faget was especially guarded. The most he would say after a year of testing was that the results were "interesting and encouraging." He had reason to hold back. While some patients showed improvements using promin, others did not. Many of the volunteers had to discontinue use of the drug because of the negative side effects. Advanced cases of the disease were slower and less likely to respond. In 1943, Faget and Pogge were still warning that it was difficult to determine how much of a patient's improved condition was due to the promin and how much was due to spontaneous remission of the disease. They did not want to create any false hopes.

Still, after two years of testing, more than half of those taking the drug had shown some improvement. They weren't cured, but the symptoms had eased. Carville's doctors concluded in 1943 that "promin appears capable of inhibiting the progress of leprosy in a considerable percentage of cases." They called the drug "the most encouraging experimental treatment" undertaken at the national leprosarium to date and "an advance in the right direction." But they were careful to add: "As yet no case of leprosy has become arrested under its influence."[13]

Testing at Carville was expanded to include other, similar drugs on the market, including diasone and promizole—all part of a group of antibiotics called sulfones. Other antibiotics, such as penicillin and streptomycin, which had shown so much success in fighting other infections, were also tried. Sister Hilary kept shooting away with her camera, tracking the results. By the time she and Dr. Faget attended the Pan-American Conference on Leprosy

in Rio de Janeiro in 1946, doctors around the world were starting to take note. Sister Hilary's photos provided strong evidence
that over time both promin and diasone produced dramatic physical improvements. The pictures she took of patients before they
were treated showed faces distorted by leprous nodules, furrowed
brows, noses bloated like cauliflower, and lips bumpy and curled.
Subsequent photos showed an almost miraculous change in some
cases, with lesions and bumps seemingly faded away, leaving little
more than what looked like a mild rash.

Faget told conferees that, after five years, half of the patients
taking the treatment were testing negative for the disease. It was
a remarkable achievement, but many doctors outside of Carville
were still not ready to declare that sulfone drugs were the treatment of choice. They believed further research was needed and
continued to rely on chaulmoogra oil. It was as though, after all
this time, they could not believe that scientists might finally be on
the right track.[14]

Though the international medical community hesitated,
patients and doctors at Carville were increasingly optimistic. Sulfone drugs weren't a cure-all, but they were proving to be a powerful weapon. Patients were being released in record numbers, three
dozen in 1946 alone. The heavy spirits at Carville began to lift like
a bayou fog. The debate was no longer whether sulfones worked,
but which one worked best. In September 1947, two patient baseball teams faced off, one called Promin, the other Diasone, in a
mock competition between the two. The Promin team won 9–5,
although both medicines continued to be used at the hospital. Each
one had its pros and cons, depending on the recipient.[15]

To the delight of patients, sulfone drugs became the treatment
of choice at Carville in 1947; the much-despised injections of chaulmoogra oil were officially stopped. "Good-by abscesses! Good-by
nausea!" declared *The Star*.[16] Surgeon General Thomas Parran Jr.

was finally prepared to declare success. "For the first time in the history of mankind, we feel that we can now say to persons who have leprosy 'There is hope.'"[17]

———

Carville's progress in the war against leprosy might have been bigger news if it hadn't been for another, much bigger, war. Residents of the isolated leprosarium were as shocked as any Americans by the attack on Pearl Harbor and just as eager to do their part. The first edition of *The Star* after the 1941 attack asked how the citizens of Carville, confined as they were, could help the troops. "The men and women in the hospital may feel that once more they are out of the mainstream of life and condemned to sit idly by while the greatest struggle in American history is going on," the paper said. But it went on to suggest there was much they could do, including learning to live with less medical help as the nation's resources were redirected to the war effort. The paper said, "Our hardest task—the one we share with every citizen of our country . . . is to stick to facts, to disregard rumors, to have courage and to share courage with our neighbors. It is easy to become an alarmist and to lose faith. You can infect others with a state of mind more easily than you can with disease."[18]

The patients took to heart the call for all Americans to chip in. They canceled the upcoming New Year's Eve celebration, and later Mardi Gras festivities, and pooled their limited resources to help fund the war effort. The Patients' Federation used $2,400 in reserve funds to buy defense bonds. They organized fairs to raise money for the American Red Cross and to buy ditty bags filled with personal items for departing soldiers. Victory gardens popped up all over the property, especially in Cottage Grove. One patient, who had immigrated from Mexico, sent the U.S. Treasury such a big donation—it's unclear how much—that he received a special government citation. "I gave my money to this country to show, in a small way, my deep appreciation for what it has done and is doing for me," the patient, Caterino Hernandez, told *The Star*.[19]

Patriotism among Carville patients was surprisingly strong, considering that the country had locked them away. Some of the healthier male patients even escaped through the hole in the fence and, as Stein wryly noted, enlisted after passing their army physicals.[20] But the irony of the patients helping in the global fight for freedom, while they were confined and unable to vote, was not lost on anyone inside the leprosarium. It was the ultimate insult, especially now that sulfone drugs had begun to show such promise. As the bacilli were increasingly being repressed in patients' bodies, the urge to rebel was swelling in their souls. The patients believed they were doing their part—"accepting" isolation in the name of protecting public health, volunteering to be subjects for medical research, and now cutting back during wartime on entertainment and more frivolous pursuits. What were they getting in return? Why were they still treated like criminals? One *Star* article in 1942 pointedly asked, "What Have We Here—Hospital or Penitentiary?"[21] Another article insisted that it was "high time that the authorities realize the folly of treating Hansen's Disease as if it were a crime instead of an illness."[22] The patients were especially offended by a column in which Dr. Faget reiterated the rules and regulations at the leprosarium, again using the language of incarceration. Individuals with Hansen's disease "may be apprehended" and "shall be detained" or "released on probation," he wrote.[23]

Faget, who had made such extraordinary advances in the medical treatment of Hansen's disease, turned out to be tone-deaf when it came to dealing with the patients' social needs. He believed that their compliance with the rules would speed recovery.[24] He wrote in *The Star* that "the careless and non-cooperating patient can through ignorance or loss of hope, harm himself by doing things detrimental to his welfare, such as dissipation and drinking." Faget warned that the "surly bird catches the germ" and that new patients should "be on guard against those old-timers" who thought they knew as much about their conditions as the doctors did.[25]

His most controversial remarks came in a 1946 column in *The Star* called "Hope Is Reborn Here," aimed at an outside audience. Public health officials believed that there were still several thousand Americans suffering from Hansen's disease who were in hiding, or in denial, because they feared being confined and ostracized. Faget encouraged them to come to Carville for treatment, especially now that there were medicines available to help them get better. But in the course of his appeal, Faget wrote that "patients live here with all the comforts of a first-class hotel" and "should consider their admission a privilege."

For those stuck behind the fence, isolated from loved ones and a normal life, these comments were over the edge. "Why do persons with leprosy not report for treatment at the National Leprosarium?" responded an indignant Stein. The answer was simple, he said. "Getting right down to the root of the problem, the majority of the patients at large will not report voluntarily because under the regulations now in effect, leprosy is regarded more as a disgrace than as a slightly communicable, bacterial disease. We doubt if many persons will accept Dr. Faget's invitation, at the cost of their freedom," he wrote. "It is very easy to get in here voluntarily but once a person signs up as a patient in the National Leprosarium, he cannot leave voluntarily." If a patient escapes, Stein said, he is likely to be hounded like a criminal and subjected to fines if "apprehended" and returned. He said people would only come to Carville willingly "when this hospital is placed on a par with hospitals for tuberculosis, admittedly a more communicable disease, and patients treated like any other sick people."[26]

Stein and the others were increasingly disturbed by their outcast status, especially now that a cure seemed near at hand. The privet hedge that separated patients and staff was a constant reminder that even those who worked at Carville did not view the people they cared for as equals, or even safe to be around. When patients went to the infirmary to see a doctor, they still had to line up in the hall outside his office and consult with him from the other side of a chain that blocked the doorway. "So whatever you told the doctor everybody else knew," one patient complained.[27] Patients and staff also had separate dining rooms, movie theaters, and post offices. They were even required to use separate entrances, and to sit in separate sections in both the Catholic and Protestant chapels.

The Daughters of Charity nurses—who had perhaps the most intimate physical contact with the patients—also preferred to keep their distance when they could, even though not one person working at the leprosarium had ever contracted the disease. When the government announced plans to build a new nurses' residence in 1940, head sister Zoe Schieswohl complained to the surgeon general that the proposal had the building extending partway onto the patients' side of the grounds. "Since leprosy is a Public Health problem and isolation of lepers compulsory in the majority of the States, we feel that it is an injustice to expect the nursing staff to live in such an area," she wrote, adding that the sisters "would much prefer to remain here in the old building than have their quarters where lepers live."[28]

One of the greatest insults came when patients tried to enjoy a quintessential American activity—drinking Coca-Cola. The local distributor refused to deliver the bottled soda to the hospital, fearing that it would destroy his business if other customers found out. The patients had friends and relatives bring the soda in for them, but the distributor refused to collect the empty bottles in exchange for a small deposit, which was the practice at the time.

So the patients got creative and, in a tiny act of rebellion, stuck their empty Coke bottles into the ground to decorate the borders of their gardens and, in one case, a gravesite. The bottles can still be seen there today.

In October of 1944 an anonymous article by "A Patient" appeared in *The Star*. Echoing President Franklin Delano Roosevelt's famous Four Freedoms speech, the writer said that those confined at Carville sought their own four freedoms—Freedom from Politics, Freedom to Hope, Freedom to Be as Other Men, and Freedom from Fear ("your unfounded fear, based on 6,000 years of mystery"). The writer concluded, "Will these freedoms be included in America's postwar plans or shall we carry on the doctrine of Hitler's 'Germanation' that 'there is no place in the State for the weak?'"[29]

The patients were clearly emboldened by the Allies' impending victory in World War II. America was on the threshold of leading the world into a new era of human rights, and Carville patients did not want to be left behind. "Don't Fence Me In," a hit tune at the time, became their unofficial anthem. The song seemed to have been written expressly for them. "Medically we had come a long way," Stein lamented. "Sociologically we were not very far removed from the days of the hand bell."[30]

While the hospital administrators expected protests from Stein and some of the other more defiant patients, it was a shock when the very proper Betty Martin weighed in. Her rage had been building as she watched friends who were discharged still being treated like pariahs, even though they no longer tested positive for the disease. Some former patients were asked to stop shopping at the local grocery store or to take their children out of the local school. A few were even run out of town by overly anxious neighbors.

It was no wonder that some of the patients who were cleared for release began to have second thoughts and consider not going home. Betty poured out their collective frustrations in the July 1945 edition of *The Star*, with a column entitled "Why Am I Not Free?" "Why am I, an American, denied my rightful heritage— LIBERTY, JUSTICE, and the PURSUIT of HAPPINESS, when my only crime is being sick?" she began her long list of questions. Why was she despised? Why was she condemned to confinement? Why was there a law that allowed her to be taken from her family? "Please, PLEASE, SOMEONE, SOMEWHERE, give me RATIONAL answers to my RATIONAL questions, or else— SET ME FREE."[31] The article resonated not only at Carville. It was reprinted in the Louisiana *Legionnaire* magazine and copies were sent to members of Congress, who contacted the surgeon general to find out what was going on down at the nation's leprosarium. Betty received letters from people around the country who expressed sympathy. Battle lines were starting to be drawn.

Johnny Harmon, now back at Carville, worked at *The Star* as both a photographer and an illustrator. He drew the cover art for that issue of the paper and perfectly captured the patients' distress. The illustration shows a Carville patient staring longingly out his window at the American flag by the front gate and, beyond that, the barbed-wire-topped fence. A John Doe letter sits on his desk. A wall calendar has the words "July 4 Independence Day, Buy Bonds for Freedom." A question mark hangs over the patient's head. The caption reads: "*. . . with liberty and justice for all.*"

Chapter 14

———————

Fighting for Freedom

IT WOULD HAVE been difficult in May of 1946 to find a more appealing and heroic couple than Hans and Gertrude Hornbostel. Hans was sixty-five, handsome and tall, a ramrod-straight army major who had survived the Bataan Death March, when the Imperial Japanese Army forced tens of thousands of American and Filipino prisoners on a brutal trek across the Philippines. His wife, Gertrude, now gray-haired and grandmotherly at fifty-two, spent the war confined by the Japanese at an internment camp in Manila.

When the couple returned to the United States after the war, Hans made a startling announcement. He told the world, from a hospital in San Francisco, that Gertrude had leprosy and he planned to go live with her at Carville—germs be damned. The *San Francisco Call-Bulletin* broke the sensational news: "S.F. Wife Leper: Army Mate Begs to Share Isolation for Life." A flood of other stories followed—"Bataan Hero Seeks Exile to Live with Leper-Wife" (*Boston Globe*); "No Greater Love Hath Any Man:

Would Be Confined with Leper Wife for Rest of Life" (*Pittsburgh Post-Gazette*); "War Hero Seeks to Join Leprosy-Stricken Wife in Exile" (*Arizona Republic*); "Mate Asks Leper's Life to Stay by Wife's Side" (*Atlanta Constitution*). The public immediately rallied in support of the couple, who were instant heroes, victims of tragedy heightened by love.

The Hornbostels had a romance straight out of Hollywood. They had met thirty-three years earlier in Guam, where she had been raised and where Hans, a marine corporal, had been sent to determine whether Gertrude's German father was a spy.[1] Instead, Hans fell in love. When her father (who Hans concluded probably was a spy) tried to prevent them from getting married, Gertrude left her home one night for a secret rendezvous with Hans. She threaded her way through mango trees and coconut palms and plunged into a river, swam downstream a half mile, then waded ashore and into her lover's arms.[2] The two were swiftly married by a navy chaplain before they set off for a life together, exploring the islands of the South Pacific, doing research for a museum, and raising three children. The Hornbostels landed in the Philippines right before the war and were soon imprisoned by the Japanese.

They now wanted to spend their remaining days together after years of separation. "Heck, I'm sixty-five. I've had my fling. I just want one other thing in life—to spend the rest of it with my wife," Hans told reporters at San Francisco's Letterman Hospital, where Gertrude was a patient in the isolation ward. The couple knew they would make a splash if they went to the media with their story. The Hornbostels invited newsreel camera crews onto the hospital grounds to record them walking arm in arm as they told their story of "deep devotion." They hoped that public pressure would make the authorities agree that they should stay together.

But the U.S. Public Health Service was unmoved. Officials said they could not allow a healthy spouse to live at Carville with sick patients. Hans could visit his wife during the day, like other spouses, but he would have to live outside the gates. Letters of protest poured into Washington. Hans appealed to an old friend, General Douglas MacArthur, who cabled his support—"I heartily endorse your desire to be with your wife"—but to no avail. Hans and Gertrude left California on a train to Louisiana in late May, disappointed but still together and smiling as they waved to reporters and photographers from the back of their railcar. Hans wore his army uniform, with four rows of ribbons. Gertrude had on a dark, brimmed hat and shaded glasses.[3]

The highly publicized case seemed like an ideal opportunity for Carville patients, who were always eager to get their story out to a broader audience. Here was a couple who publicly embraced Hansen's disease, dismissing the stigma and fear of contagion as meaningless. Instead, the initial news coverage of the Hornbostels' case was a public relations disaster, as far as the patients were concerned. They were angry and upset when they gathered around a bulletin board outside *The Star*'s office and read the latest news clippings shortly before the Hornbostels arrived.[4] Many of the stories perpetuated the myths and prejudices that the patients had been trying so hard to correct. The newspapers made it seem as if Gertrude were doomed, even though she had an extremely mild case of the disease and some doctors thought there was a good chance she could be cured. "Facing her is a life of virtual imprisonment in a federal leprosarium, while the disease completes its ravages of face and body," read one article, which ignored the fact that her only symptom so far was numbness in her hands.[5] Almost every newspaper called her a "leper" or, worse, a "leper wife." One paper described Carville as "that dark place which brings to mind that ominous word 'unclean.'"[6] Many articles attributed the disease to the "filthy Jap camp" where Gertrude had been confined, even though she had likely picked up the germ years earlier.

Stanley Stein, Betty Martin, and others on the *Star* staff decided some quick damage control was needed. They were especially angry at the California doctor who was quoted in the newspapers as saying that Gertrude's chances for recovery were "that of a snowball in hell." The doctor also said that Hans's chance of getting the disease were "100%," which was not even remotely true. Stein and the others collected their spare change and headed to the canteen, where the telephone was mounted on the wall, and started to make calls. They tried to contact the California doctor to set the record straight, but he denied making the comments. Stein then called the United Press newswire office to get someone to correct the misinformation in the UP's reports. He also invited a local reporter to come see for himself that Carville was not a place of doom. Stein told the reporter that stories depicting the leprosarium as such were misleading. "Such things make people believe this place is the end of hope. Actually, it is the beginning," he said. Stein noted that doctors had made tremendous progress using sulfone drugs and that a cure for Hansen's disease appeared within reach.[7] *The Star* ran an editorial before the Hornbostels arrived, criticizing the couple for creating a media frenzy. It said that patients were filled with "anger, resentment and amazement at all this hullabaloo."[8]

The Hornbostels quickly realized that things had gotten out of hand and tried to get their message back on track. They knew better than most people that leprosy was barely contagious, because they had lived for so many years in the South Pacific, where the disease was far more common than in the United States and more widely accepted as part of life. Hans complained to reporters that he had publicized his wife's case intending to enlighten people about Hansen's disease but that the newspapers had turned it into a "melodramatic mess."[9] When the couple finally arrived at Carville, Hans tried to set the record straight.

He told the newsmen who greeted them that "people have a foolish dread" of Hansen's disease. He even said that he was grateful
his wife had leprosy rather than a more serious illness, such as
cancer, tuberculosis, or syphilis.

Gertrude then wrote an article for *The Star* called "As I See
It."[10] She blamed public health officials for the controversy. By
segregating patients, they were keeping "alive the fear and horror
which they should be the first ones to help to dispel. . . . There is
no reason why we should not have public dispensaries all over the
country where people could get treatment or why private practi-
tioners should not be allowed 'officially' to treat patients." Gertrude said the government had a responsibility to inform the public
about the minimal risk of contracting leprosy. It all came back to
the Bible, she wrote. "I think it suits the health authorities to be
able to carry over from biblical times the hush-hush attitude which
makes outcasts of free-born Americans, herds them into stock-
ades and deprives them of the right to come and go as they please."
The woman who once ran through the jungle to be with her lover
appeared to like making waves as much as Early and Stein.

The Hornbostels turned out to be "our kind of people," said
Stein, who realized the case could now be used to the patients'
advantage.[11] It was a perfect example of how much more the public
needed to learn about Hansen's disease. Hans told reporters that
he was shocked to discover that Carville patients were treated like
prisoners. "My wife had a fence around her in the Philippines. And
now her own people put one around her here," he said. The Hornbostels were also disturbed to learn that Gertrude would lose her
right to vote. "It's the most damnable thing I ever heard of. The
state of Louisiana is treating these intelligent, good American people like so many criminals or insane," said Hans.[12]

The patients, with the help of the American Legion, had been
pushing for years to regain their right to vote, which was denied

them by a Louisiana law prohibiting those under state care from casting ballots. But the national news coverage of the Hornbostels' complaints made all the difference. The voting ban was difficult to justify for those who had survived such hardship during the war. Just one day after Hans's remarks, a state senator introduced a bill allowing Carville patients to vote. The legislation was quickly passed and Louisiana voters that November overwhelmingly approved a constitutional amendment allowing the change to go into effect. One politically active patient, Fred Smith, was especially thrilled. He had snuck through the hole in the fence to cast his ballot in five previous elections, which had resulted in at least two stints in the Carville jail.[13]

Hans was not allowed to live with his wife, but he quickly became a prominent fixture at the hospital. He rented a room two miles down the road in a house he shared with three Carville employees and the wife of another patient. Every morning, Hans rode his bicycle to the leprosarium and entered through the front gate, greeting the guards, doctors, and everyone else he saw with an exuberant "Good morning." He and Gertrude spent their days together at the little house she was able to secure in Cottage Grove. They worked in their garden, cooked meals, and played with their two black Scotties. Hans became active in the Carville American Legion post and gave speeches to outside groups to correct public misperceptions about Hansen's disease. It was almost like a normal retiree's life. Except that at seven each night, Hans had to leave and go back to his rented room. Patients later said, however, that he would sometimes sneak right back through the hole in the fence and spend the night with his wife. He would then crawl back out early the next morning and reenter through the front gate, cheerfully greeting the guards—a ruse that likely fooled few.[14]

Gertrude spent her spare time answering the thousands of letters she received from supporters across the country. She also wrote articles for *The Star*, some of which received outside press coverage. Gertrude did not hold back. She made clear how disturbed she was by the way American society treated leprosy victims. In one article, she complained that public health officials "don't seem to be endowed with the imagination to put themselves in our place. They look at the patient from the professional standpoint only, wearing blinders to the fact that we too have human urges and feelings."[15]

The patients were starting to attract more national attention, thanks in large part to the Hornbostels and the end of the war. Newspaper reporters from around the country were suddenly interested in the curious little hospital in southern Louisiana, and in a disease that many Americans believed had been eradicated ages ago. An Associated Press story in June of 1946 tried to dispel some of the most common myths. The article ran in dozens of papers under headlines such as "Experts Say Leprosy Isn't Hopeless Evil," "Leprosy Found Overrated," "New Drugs Help to Halt Leprosy," and "Leprosy Less Infectious Than T.B., Smallpox." It was just the kind of publicity that Stein and the other patient-activists craved. In August, a correspondent and photographer from *Life* magazine came to the hospital and spent five days interviewing and photographing patients as they went about their daily lives.[16] The aim was to show that the disease was not as brutal as most people believed. The patients were disappointed to learn later that the story would not be published. The magazine editors said the photos were not up to their standards, although Stein speculated that the patients probably looked too healthy to make for a sensational story.[17]

But that was a minor setback. Patients who had been reluctant before to expose themselves to the outside world started to welcome visitors at the hospital so they could share their stories. They were inspired in part by a visit from Helen Keller, who had overcome her blindness and deafness to become a successful author and political activist. She arrived with her longtime companion, Polly Thompson, both of them wearing small hats covered in flowers. Keller praised the patients for their "indomitable faith" in confronting challenges similar to her own.[18]

The patients lobbied hospital administrators to open up the grounds to more guests, and even organized a group of residents to give tours.[19] In 1946, Carville had a record 5,707 visitors—doctors, nurses, veterans, journalists, and curious citizens.[20] One visitor was I. T. Kelly from the Nebraska-based Railway Educational Bureau, which trained rail workers who might one day have to transport leprosy patients to the hospital. Kelly told *The Star* that "wild horses could not have dragged me into this place without the recent widespread publicity . . . showing that it is just as safe to visit this institution as it would be to visit any other hospital in the United States."[21]

The patients had never before received so much positive attention. They were certain they were getting closer to freedom. Johnny Harmon drew an illustration for the cover of the September 1946 issue of *The Star* that captured their excitement—and amusement—at suddenly being the center of attraction. The picture shows the hospital courtyard filled with people, including reporters from *Life* magazine and the Associated Press, legionnaires from New York, and patients and doctors giving tours. "Why doctor, they look just like real people," comments one of the visitors in the cartoon. "But aren't you afraid to work here?" another visitor asks a guide. "I'm a patient," the guide responds.[22]

On a Sunday afternoon that September, the national American Legion Auxiliary helped the patients take another step forward. Dozens of auxiliary members, patients, and hospital personnel gathered around the patients' baseball diamond as the auxiliary presented Carville with two 1946 Buick Super station wagons.

The cars were elegant, with sleek wood siding, whitewall tires, and shiny metal grilles, which would soon become dusty from traveling along the unpaved roads outside. One car was to be used for picking up visiting family members and friends at a nearby railway station. The other was to take patients back home for authorized visits. Because leprosy patients were still not allowed to use public transportation, finding a way home was often such a challenge that many opted not to go, even when granted a leave.

But the first trip was for neither purpose. A group of patients piled into one of the new station wagons and took a two-hour ride around the nearby countryside. Some of them had not been outside the hospital gates in twenty years.[23]

There were other signs that Carville was finally opening up. The stands at the baseball field filled that summer with spectators who came to watch the patients' fast-pitch softball team play against several local teams. It was the beginning of what would become known as the River League. The Carville All Stars won their first game against the Louisiana Creamery from Baton Rouge, and ended the season with six wins, eight losses, and a tie—although for the patients, every game they played as part of the community league was seen as a victory.[24]

Things were clearly changing for the better, both socially and medically. Besides a record number of discharges in 1946, the number of deaths was so low that a patient who worked as a grave digger in Carville's cemetery complained that he didn't have enough to do.[25]

The good news became personal that year for Harry and Betty Martin. Harry's ulcers had healed, the swelling in his hands and feet had gone down, and he was starting to get a string of negative monthly test results. Their excitement grew as Betty started to see negative results as well. In December, Betty had her tenth negative in a row, and Harry had his twelfth, which meant the unthinkable had finally happened. He was free to go. That night, Betty, Harry, and a few of their friends gathered in Stein's cottage, Wits' End, to celebrate with a toast. But the couple's joy was tempered because they had to wait at least two more months to be truly free, since Harry refused to leave without Betty. Neither of them told their families that they were so close to being discharged, for fear of getting their hopes up. They didn't want to jinx things now. While they nervously waited for the next two tests, Harry took a job driving one of the new station wagons, which gave him some practice behind the wheel, a skill he would need when—if—he and Betty were allowed to leave.[26]

Christmas at Carville that year was especially joyous. The war was over, there was hope in the air, and many outsiders were eager to help the patients celebrate. The female employees of a Chicago telephone company, the Delta Sigma Epsilon sorority, the American Legion Auxiliary, the Tulane Housing Project, and others donated food, decorations, and piles of gifts for the patients, especially for the children. Everyone at the leprosarium gathered on December 22 in the recreation center ballroom, which had been transformed into a Christmas wonderland, with decorated trees, poinsettias, and strings of colored lights. There were homemade cookies, eggnog, and piles of candy. Major Hornbostel, dressed as Santa Claus, distributed gifts, and a group of young dancers from Baton Rouge entertained the crowd. At one point, legionnaire Louis L. McCormick, an active supporter of the patients, got up on stage and took the microphone. He said that he had just returned from a meeting in Washington, where a new Advisory Committee on Leprosy had made some yet-to-be-announced recommendations to the Public Health Service about how to improve conditions at Carville. He would not reveal the recommendations, but he gave the patients a hint. "You have every reason to be in high good humor," he said.

That New Year's Eve an orchestra from the nearby town of Lafayette played music as the patients danced well past midnight. "And so 1947 has come to Carville," one of them wrote the following day. "We feel confident that at long last the sun is to shine on us in this horseshoe bend of the Father of Waters as it has never shone before."[27]

Chapter 15

Not Bright Enough

STEIN AND SOME of the others did not think the sun was shining brightly enough. Conditions had improved, but patients were still denied basic rights and the freedom to come and go as they chose.

Frustrated that things were not changing with the speed they wanted, the patients had formed a lobbying group at the end of 1945 called the United Patients' Committee for Social Improvement and Rehabilitation, which included members of the Patients' Federation, the *Star* staff, and the American Legion post. The committee came up with a fifteen-point plan to improve the lives of those isolated at Carville and gave it to the Advisory Committee on Leprosy, which had been named by the surgeon general to propose how the government could change the way it handled Hansen's disease.

Among the patients' recommendations, first and foremost, was getting rid of forced confinement. They proposed that outpatient clinics be opened around the country where those with Hansen's disease could be treated closer to home. The patient committee also recommended that the government give financial assistance to the dependents of those at Carville who had been their family's sole breadwinner, that living quarters be provided for married couples, and that the terms *abscond* and *parole* be stricken from hospital regulations. They also suggested that the government do more to educate the public about Hansen's disease so that people would be less fearful of those who had it. It was an ambitious agenda, but the patients were hopeful that the Advisory Committee would adopt their recommendations. The government panel included several allies, such as Sister Catherine and American Legion officials, along with public health and medical experts. But the patients did not leave anything to chance. They typed up their demands and sent a copy to each member of the Advisory Committee.[1]

The patients' campaign ran into opposition right from the start, but on a very surprising front. Iberville Parish residents, who had once opposed the leprosarium, were now worried that it might shut down if the patients got their way and were allowed to leave. Carville provided hundreds of well-paying government jobs—cooks, groundskeepers, maintenance workers, orderlies—as well as business for local merchants. The leprosarium also brought international prestige to a community that was otherwise poor and easily forgotten. Residents were proud that doctors from all over the world came to their isolated part of the state.

Stein complained that "guerrillas" from nearby towns—Carville, Gonzales, and St. Gabriel, where many hospital employees lived—were trying to sabotage the patients' efforts. Street signs directing outside visitors to the leprosarium mysteriously disappeared. Letters were sent to the Baton Rouge Chamber of Commerce ominously predicting that the city could be "overrun with lepers" if patients were given more freedom to leave the grounds. Local legionnaires also received complaints that the United Patients' Committee did not represent the majority of Carville's residents but rather a small, disgruntled faction. The committee responded by getting almost all 370 patients to sign a petition saying they did in fact support the committee's work.

The main issue appeared to be the 25–50 percent "hazard pay" that employees received on top of their regular wages for working at the leprosarium. The workers feared they would lose that extra pay if the public believed that leprosy was only mildly contagious. The patients, on the other hand, found even the name *hazard pay* highly offensive. They argued that it only perpetuated the myth that leprosy posed a serious threat to the public.

Relations between the patients and nearby residents became especially strained over the patients' demand that they be allowed to vote. Residents worried that hospital voters might dominate local politics in the sparsely populated region. While the constitutional amendment restoring the patients' right to vote passed statewide by a wide margin—72,696 to 20,158—the towns of Carville and St. Gabriel opposed it by a vote of 103 to 18. When the local registrar came to the hospital to sign up the new voters, he insisted that they use their real names and former places of residence, something many of the patients were reluctant to do. They had assumed aliases at Carville to avoid exposing their families to embarrassment and rejection back home. But many of them finally relented and registered.

As some parish residents had feared, the hospital became a powerful voting bloc and an important campaign stop for state and local politicians.[2] Those looking for votes often came on movie nights, when the patients gathered in the theater. But the candidates had only a few minutes to speak. They were warned they would lose more votes than they'd win if they delayed the start of the movie. Some candidates also brought gifts, such as sugar, Creole sausage, bicycles, and beer to woo the Carville electorate.[3]

The conflict between the patients and the community came

to a head when a rumor began circulating that a female patient had been taken in one of the new station wagons to a local beauty parlor to get her hair done, sending other customers fleeing into the streets. The rumor was so widespread that it made its way to Public Health Service officials in Washington, who demanded to know from Dr. Faget, who was still in charge, what was going on. Stein also received a letter from a legionnaire in Arkansas who had heard the report and advised the newspaper editor to recognize that "the rights of others must be respected." Faget decided he needed to quell the unrest. He sent a staff member out to collect signed affidavits from all of the local salon owners confirming that no Carville patient had been a customer and that the rumored incident had never occurred.[4]

Throughout it all, the Advisory Committee on Leprosy considered the patients' recommendations, and in late December 1946— as legionnaire McCormick hinted at the Christmas party—it endorsed many of them, though not all. It proposed a more liberal leave policy for patients, financial aid for the families of breadwinners, and the opening of regional diagnostic and treatment centers.[5] The patients were ecstatic. But with the exception of the proposal that patients be allowed up to one month of leave twice a year, with a doctor's approval, few of the items on the list were adopted by the Public Health Service. "Practically nothing has been accomplished of the numerous other recommendations made," the Daughters of Charity lamented in their annals.[6]

One obstacle was that, more than sixty years after the start of the Louisiana Leper Home, U.S. health officials were still surprisingly divided over how serious a threat leprosy posed. Dr. George McCoy, one of the nation's leading leprologists, wrote in 1940 that "it seems reasonably clear" that segregating patients "has had no appreciable influence in restricting the spread of leprosy." It was a stunning admission about a policy the government had pursued for decades. But in 1950, the doctor in charge of leprosy at the Public Health Service's Communicable Disease Center—which would eventually become the Centers for Disease Control and Prevention—expressed the opposite opinion. Lucius Badger said he did not believe that leprosy was "barely" contagious at all and he argued for maximum isolation of those who had the disease.[7] In the absence of scientific certainty over exactly how Hansen's disease was spread, the safest course of action appeared to be doing what had always been done—keeping the victims confined. There was also a feeling among some in Washington that the patients at Carville had become too outspoken and needed to be reined in.

The patients were not about to stop pushing for change, no matter what the doctors said, and they were encouraged by an old friend. Sister Catherine visited Carville in December of 1946, days before the Christmas party, and addressed patients gathered in the movie theater. Still wearing her starched white cornette with its uplifted wings, Sister Catherine commanded everyone's attention, and she did not mince words. She told the patients that they had "a date with destiny" and should not be so quick to accept their fate. "If I have a fault to find with you, it is that you fail to grasp the great role that is yours. Is it a small thing that you have an opportunity to change world opinion, to challenge 6,000-year-old opinions, to alter universal practices?" she asked. "In your hands rests the fate . . . of every sufferer from Hansen's disease throughout the world, and of all those destined henceforth to bear the burden of the disease."[8] Echoing the words of British prime minister Winston Churchill, she asked the spellbound patients, "Will it be said of you: 'Never in the medical history of the world have so many owed so much to so few'?"

Sister Catherine believed that the only way to eradicate leprosy was to educate the public. She said victims were unlikely to come forward for treatment as long as they faced "social ostracism, unjust confinement, separation from loved ones, frustrations of lawful ambitions, denial of inherent human rights." In a show of solidarity with the patients, she called herself one of them: "Hansen's Disease merely makes us patients. Ignorance makes us victims."[9] She urged the patients to tell their stories to the world.

Among those inspired by the speech was Betty Martin. On February 3, 1947, Betty went to get her twelfth monthly skin test. The possibility that it might be negative, and that she would be free to go, was almost too much for her to bear. She tried to relax as the technician took two skin smears for testing, and she went back to *The Star*'s office to keep herself busy while waiting for the results. Harry was not so calm. He returned to the lab repeatedly until the results were ready. When they were, he rushed to give his wife the news. The test was negative. They could finally leave Carville together. Betty tried to continue typing as she absorbed the incredible news, but her hands began to shake. Before long, she and Harry were surrounded by friends, who offered their congratulations. Betty and Harry could now tell their parents and start planning for the future. Betty could also finally kiss her nephew, the little boy she had avoided touching when she was home so many years before and who was now a young man.[10]

For the next few months Harry and Betty were treated to a round of parties as they prepared for their transition to a new life. They met with reporters from the *St. Louis Post-Dispatch*, *Collier's* magazine, and other publications to tell their story. They were among several patients interviewed for the popular *We the People* radio program, which was broadcast from the Carville movie theater before a crowd of five hundred patients, personnel, and visitors that summer.[11]

Finally, the big day came. Betty had trouble sleeping and was up early that morning to get ready. She made herself a café au lait and drank it in her room alone before going out to meet Harry, who was waiting in a car outside. In the past, some patients had been sent off to freedom with a line of sisters waving farewell with their handkerchiefs, or escorted to the gate by other patients with flowers as if "risen from the dead"—a symbolic undoing of the ritual medieval burial service.[12] But the Martins wanted to leave without making a scene. After all these years, it was hard enough to go without teary goodbyes. When the couple approached the front gate, though, the guard asked them to wait. The new medical officer in charge, Dr. Frederick Johansen—or Dr. Jo, as the patients called him—had something to give them. The doctor and his wife came out to present the Martins with their official discharge papers. They were among the first to get a new version of the government forms. They were not identified as "lepers" who were "no longer a menace to public health." Instead, the certificates gave the reason for discharge as "No further treatment necessary." With that parting gift, the Martins were off.

———

Dr. Jo had taken over after Dr. Faget had had a heart attack earlier that year and been transferred to a less stressful job at the U.S. Marine Hospital in New Orleans. One morning in July, around the same time the Martins were leaving Carville, Faget's body was found below his fifth-floor office window. It's not clear what happened, but the hospital's chief doctor speculated that the fifty-six-year-old had felt another heart attack coming on, leaned out the window to get some fresh air, and fallen to his death. *The Star* called Faget, the man whose curiosity had led to a discovery that would eventually affect millions of lives, a "true scientist, one who did not consider established methods as perfect and permanent, but as essentially incomplete."[13]

Dr. Jo was a different kind of pioneer. He turned out to be one of the patients' strongest allies yet and, as Stein said, made "a crack in the penal-type attitude" at Carville.[14] One of the first things Johansen did was to remove the three strands of barbed wire that ran along the top of the chain-link fence that surrounded the complex. The gravel road over which so many patients and visitors had traveled uncomfortably for years was finally paved. The leprosarium also got its own post-office substation, although the mail was still sterilized. Most important, Dr. Jo agreed that patients could be discharged without necessarily having twelve monthly negative test results in a row, as long as doctors determined they could safely be cared for at home. Local health authorities would also have to approve and the patients' families would have to pay for their care.

For patients, it was a good start, but they wanted more. One of the benefits of getting healthier was that they now had more energy to lobby for change and more incentive to question their treatment. Stein spent hours writing advertisers, encyclopedia publishers, news organizations, and others to correct common misstatements about Hansen's disease. At one point, he contacted the creator of the popular *Rex Morgan, M.D.* comic strip after Morgan was shown pointing to another character and saying, "You're treating her like a leper!" Not only did the creator, psychiatrist Nicholas Dallis, apologize to Stein, but future episodes of the comic strip featured Carville and illustrated some of the obstacles faced by people with Hansen's disease.[15]

The patients became increasingly outspoken. In the March 1947 issue of *The Star*, an anonymous patient—using the pseudonym "Key Pitt" for a column called "Under Your Hat"—complained that doctors sometimes took advantage of patients in experimental drug tests. The writer said that patients were willing to cooperate but that the administration "[hung] cooperation over their heads like the Sword of Damocles," as though it were a condition for getting more freedom and privileges. "Permission to take a deep breath is always preceded by a lecture on cooperation and followed by the admonition that 'as long as everyone behaves we believe in giving as much freedom as possible.'" The writer went on to note that in one recent test, some patients were given a different drug from the one they had agreed to take and began to suffer negative reactions. The writer said that "the unfortunate victims of this unprincipled deception are numerous and seriously demoralized. . . . The spirit of cooperation has been seriously threatened and unless there is some honest explanation and precaution against the carelessness that is becoming increasingly evident in our laboratory it may be lost forever."[16]

It was not the only time the patients pushed back against being used as test subjects. A few months earlier, Gertrude Hornbostel responded to Faget's declaration that patients should consider admission to the hospital "a privilege" by writing in *The Star*, "It seems to me that the doctors in this hospital are the 'privileged,' as they are the only ones in this country who have the opportunity to experiment on patients with Hansen's disease." Hornbostel argued that a cure for leprosy would have been discovered much sooner if patients had not been isolated from major medical centers, where research would be more robust.[17]

The patients got a morale boost in February of 1948 when one of the first big-time entertainers came to the leprosarium to perform. Popular actor and ventriloquist Edgar Bergen arrived with his sidekick puppet, Charlie McCarthy, and his wife, Frances, and they were treated like royalty. Patients and staff laid out a red carpet and lined up outside the recreation center to greet their famous guests. Bergen was also presented with an oversize key to the grounds, which one patient quipped wasn't a key to get into Carville, but one Bergen could use "to let us out."[18] The famous ventriloquist said he hoped his appearance would encourage other performers to visit, so "then gradually the stigma that is erroneously tacked on to the poor folks who have this disease may be partially dissipated."[19]

Several months after Bergen's visit, the patients got another high-profile ally in their effort to change public perception. Joey Guerrero, a Filipina who had spied for the United States during the Japanese occupation of the Philippines, was admitted to the hospital amid great fanfare. Patients waited for hours on the front steps of the infirmary to greet Guerrero and to present her with a big bouquet of red roses. In her room, they had draped a banner woven in the colors of the Philippine flag—red, yellow, and blue— with the words "Welcome Joey."

Guerrero was not just any patient. She was a war hero who had been given the United States' highest civilian award, the Medal of Freedom, extremely rare for someone who was not a U.S. citizen. Guerrero had used her leprosy to help the Allies recapture Manila. The Japanese were terrified of the disease and their soldiers generally left Guerrero alone as she moved around the city mapping out the locations of gun defenses to leak to the Americans. In 1944, she snuck across enemy lines to give a map of mines planted in Manila Bay to the approaching U.S. forces. With that action, she was credited with saving the lives of hundreds of Americans, including detainees such as Gertrude Hornbostel. But after the war, Guerrero ended up in a squalid leprosarium in the Philippines. Her supporters were eventually able to get the U.S. government to allow her to come to Carville, even though the hospital was supposed to be reserved for American citizens.[20] When she arrived, Guerrero said she was thrilled to be in "a happy energetic community teeming with life," where there were dinner parties, movies, and plays.[21] She soon joined the Hornbostels, Stein, and *The Star* in the campaign to educate the public about Hansen's disease. Guerrero, with her heroic story, was a welcome addition to the team.

After three years at Carville, Gertrude Hornbostel had had enough. In the summer of 1949 she wrote in *The Star* that she would not be living there if she had a choice. She said that the hot, humid climate was hurting, not helping, her recovery. Gertrude also complained about the complete lack of privacy when patients had to consult a doctor in front of a roomful of other patients, and noted that on one occasion a newspaper reporter was allowed to sit in on a patient consultation. "Should a patient's private affairs, feelings and personal symptoms become public property, to be bandied about the grounds of this institution and in the country's press?" she asked. Gertrude essentially accused Carville's doctors of violating their Hippocratic Oath to, among other things, respect their patients' privacy.[22]

The article caused a furor, especially in Washington. *The Star* by this time had thousands of subscribers around the country. The Forty and Eight veterans' group, an offshoot of the American Legion, had adopted the paper as a national project and actively solicited subscriptions from its members. The Public Health Service knew its reputation was at stake. Stein added to the controversy by writing an editorial supporting Gertrude's complaints.

Top officials in the Public Health Service thought that the Carville rabble-rousers were getting out of control. This was a time when some in the government, including the House Un-American Activities Committee, were intent on rooting out subversives. It was not good to question authority too much. It's not clear exactly what happened, but an unidentified individual seems to have been assigned to work undercover at *The Star* and to report back to Washington about the newspaper and its influence. In an unsigned and undated report—which remains in Public Health Service files today—the investigator questioned whether Stein truly represented the majority of Carville's patients. "Among the patients there are two schools of thought on *The Star*. They like it or they don't," the writer said, adding that Stein "is influenced most effectively from the outside, by the professional do-gooders who worship him." The report's author raised the possibility of turning the patient newspaper into a "company organ" that would come out only four times a year with "no stories and allusions to friction between the patients and staff, the patients and the Public Health Service."[23] As much as the health service might have wanted to stifle Stein, those changes were never made. Dr. Jo, a staunch ally of the patients, resisted. He also reminded the patients that they were free to ask for private consultations with their doctors if they chose to do so.

Three months after her controversial column ran in *The Star*, Gertrude Hornbostel was discharged and moved with her husband to a little cottage on Long Island in New York. Another troublesome patient was gone.

———

While some things had changed, many remained the same. Early one morning in March of 1949, a fourteen-year-old girl in Corpus Christi, Texas, was taken away from her parents, her seven siblings, and the only home she had ever known. The girl had been diagnosed with Hansen's disease and an armed deputy sheriff and nurse came to her house to drive her to Carville. "They kidnapped me from right under their eyes because when my mother and father reached out to hug me goodbye, the nurse pushed them away, and I'll never forgive her for that," she said many years later. The girl's Mexican American parents, who did not speak English, thought that their daughter was being taken to a nearby hospital for treatment. It would take several days before they learned the truth.[24]

The girl was put in the back seat of a car, most likely a big station wagon that the Texas health department routinely used to round up its leprosy patients. Two older women were already there, sitting on a tarp. The trip to Louisiana was long and uncomfortable. When the three patients were allowed out to use a bathroom, the nurse followed them with rubber gloves and a bottle of rubbing alcohol to clean up after they were done. When they stopped for meals, the patients ate in the car, on paper plates with plastic utensils, while the nurse and driver ate inside the restaurant.

When she finally reached Carville and was admitted, the young girl—who had no idea where she was or what was happening to her—cried herself to sleep. "I would ask when I was going to go home, and they kept telling me, 'within six months.'" She ended up staying at Carville for eleven years, and then returning later for another twenty. Back in Corpus Christi, the girl's school burned her desk and all of her books—as officials had done more than two decades earlier when two schoolboys with leprosy were identified in Newark, New Jersey. When the Texas girl eventually received a pass to visit her family, a large "Quarantine" sign was posted outside their house.

This happened in 1949, four years after the American Public Health Association recommended against isolating those with Hansen's disease, eight years after doctors at Carville started using promin, and decades after some in the medical community insisted that treating leprosy patients like outcasts was cruel, unnecessary, and counterproductive.[25]

Chapter 16

———◦◦———

"It's Tallulah, Darling"

ON A SUNDAY afternoon in August 1950, Stein was called up to the administration building to take a long-distance call from New York. He thought it might be the Hornbostels, who still kept in touch with their old friend. Or it might be his cousin, who also lived in New York. When he picked up the phone and heard a husky voice say, "It's Tallulah, darling," Stein almost fainted. He was an ardent fan of the flamboyant actress Tallulah Bankhead, one of Broadway's biggest stars at the time. He repeatedly played a recording of her performance in the play *The Little Foxes*, just to hear her speak. For a blind man who loved the theater, the sound of Bankhead's "warm, dark contralto" was priceless.[1] To hear her voice over the phone was unimaginable.

Stein and Bankhead had a mutual friend, Joy Lamont, the wife of a Hollywood producer. Lamont knew that Stein was a huge admirer of Bankhead and had arranged for the call. The two spoke for almost an hour, Stein telling the actress how much he admired her work, and Bankhead introducing Stein over the phone to some of her houseguests that day. They included sculptor Lillian Greneker, who was in the process of making a bronze bust of Bankhead. The actress told Stein that she would send him a papier mâché copy when it was completed. She also promised him that she would visit Carville the next time she came to New Orleans for work.[2]

Stein was in heaven after he put down the phone. "It will take a high-flying plane to bring me down to earth," he wrote Bankhead the following day. "But who wants to come down? . . . . Never, even in one of my wildest flights of fancy (and I have many), did I dream that I would be talking with warmth and intimacy with you."[3]

Thus began a most unusual relationship between the blind leprosy patient and the internationally acclaimed actress. While Stein was certainly starstruck, he was also keenly aware that Bankhead could provide a useful platform to promote the Carville story he wanted so much to get to the outside world. The star was famous for her sometimes outrageous and scandalous behavior, including heavy drinking and multiple love affairs. But she was also known for adopting seemingly lost causes. She came from a political family; her father had been a longtime Democratic congressman from Alabama and served as Speaker of the House. Embracing the forgotten victims of Hansen's disease was right up her alley.

Bankhead invited Stein to come visit her in New York whenever he was able to get a medical pass from the hospital. But Stein was nervous about leaving Carville after all these years, even for a short visit. It was a sign of how confinement could undermine someone's confidence to such a degree that the man who was so assertive seeking freedom for others was reluctant to take advantage of it himself. Stein told Bankhead that he'd take a rain check, noting that the disease had left his hands "badly crippled and this is embarrassing to me—well, you can understand."[4] Bankhead insisted, saying that her invitation was sincere. "When you came

into my life I kind of got my second wind. I never leaned on anyone or anything in my life—but if I ever did it would be on you,"
she wrote shortly after their first call. "So when I said 'come up' I
meant—'come up.' "[5]

Bankhead continued to call Stein for months and to introduce
him over the phone to her Broadway friends. She also sent him an
early Christmas present, not a copy but the actual bronze bust of
herself. When Stein protested that it was too generous a gift, especially for someone who could not see, she responded, "But you can
feel it, darling. You can appreciate my bone structure."[6]

As Stein had suspected, Bankhead proved extremely helpful
in getting the patients' message out to a wider audience. Like an
aggressive saleswoman, she persuaded dozens of her Broadway
and Hollywood friends to subscribe to *The Star*, and she insisted
that they sign up for five years rather than one. Big-name celebrities
at the time, such as José Ferrer, Perry Como, Ed Wynn, Jimmy
Durante, Marlene Dietrich, Ginger Rogers, and Ray Middleton,
sent Stein five dollars each for their subscriptions, telling him that
Bankhead had encouraged them to do so. Stein responded to each
with a letter of thanks, an invitation to visit Carville, and a request
that they use their influence to correct any falsehoods they heard
about Hansen's disease. "As you will see by reading *The Star* our
problems are largely those of public attitude," Stein wrote to José
Ferrer in a typical letter. "The general public has not yet become
sufficiently informed about Hansen's disease nor sufficiently interested in its problems."[7]

Stein also knew how to butter up his new fans. He drafted
a sample letter for an assistant at *The Star* to send to Bankhead's
"big shot friends." He even suggested where the assistant could
insert what Stein called the "I saw you last night at Carnegie Hall
and your playing sent itsy-bitsy wiggles of joy up and down my
spine" paragraph.[8] He was well aware that flattery was an easy

way to keep such big-name backers on board. By May, Bankhead had signed up more than forty high-profile subscribers. If the Public Health Service wanted to rein in the patient newspaper now, they'd have to do it in the glare of a much brighter spotlight.

Carville was also attracting a lot more attention on another front. Betty Martin had followed Sister Catherine's advice, and after her discharge wrote a memoir about life at the leprosarium. Her book, *Miracle at Carville*, was released by Doubleday in late 1950 and quickly became a best seller. It was chosen the following year to be a *Reader's Digest* selection, exposing many Americans for the first time to the Louisiana leprosarium and the way patients were stigmatized. A reviewer for the *Los Angeles Times* said the book was impossible to put down. "It is a thrilling story and Betty Martin, which is not her real name, as she still hides her identity, wrote it partly in protest to the mistaken notions surrounding an illness which makes social outcasts of its innocent victims." The reviewer called the book "fascinating and rewarding, never morbid, and filled with a hardy spiritual courage."[9] Still, to the annoyance of the Carville patients, the headline on the review called Martin "a woman leper." While public sympathies appeared to be shifting, there was a lot of educating left to do.

One of the great ironies of Martin's success was that she was unable to enjoy her fame. She and Harry lived in constant fear that people would discover their secret past. After they left the leprosy hospital, they went back to using their real names. Edwina Parra could not admit that she was the best-selling author Betty Martin.

Hollywood also seemed eager to get in on the Carville story. Columbia Pictures announced plans to make a movie about Hansen's disease based on a book by Perry Burgess called *Who Walk Alone*, about a Spanish-American War veteran who ended up at the Culion colony in the Philippines. The movie company planned to change the story and focus instead on the fictional tale of a World

War II veteran admitted to Carville. The excitement level was high along the Mississippi when the patients gathered in the recreation building in late 1949 to hear producer William Dozier describe the project. Among those rumored to be under consideration for the lead role were actors Montgomery Clift, Mel Ferrer, and Dana Andrews. "We are conscious of the real responsibility we have in bringing a story about Hansen's disease to the screen," Dozier told the patients.[10] But that was the last they saw of him. A few months later, the *Hollywood Reporter* wrote that "Columbia is having trouble getting a crew for its leprosy picture because the shooting involves entering a leprosarium in Louisiana—and the lads are scared."[11] Columbia denied that this was the case and said crew members were excited about the project, but the company later dropped its option to produce the film. It blamed recent box-office failures involving disease-related movies, especially *Panic in the Streets*, which had been released earlier that year. That movie was about a Public Health Service doctor trying to stop the spread of the plague in New Orleans. Stein was not convinced. "I think it was the same old leprophobia bugaboo which scared them off," he told his friend Lamont.[12]

Still, Carville and the fate of its patients was turning into something of a cause célèbre for the entertainment world. Stein received at least two handwritten letters in 1951 from one of Lamont's other famous friends, a young actor named Marlon Brando, who had recently won widespread praise for his performance as Stanley Kowalski in *A Streetcar Named Desire* on Broadway. The twenty-seven-year-old Brando wrote Stein that Lamont had filled him in about Carville and he wanted to help. "She told me many moving things about you and the life of the people there," Brando scrawled in an awkward but earnest three-page note. "The grossness that comes as a result of a twisted and gnarled impression of people with Hansen's disease, to me, is bitterly unfortunate and I wish you would write me and tell me how I might be of service to you and others who are affected with the embarrassing social stigma of being misunderstood. If I can be of assistance, please write me. . . . Sincerely Yours, Marlon Brando."[13]

"Dear Marlon Brando: Your name immediately rang a bell," Stein responded, adding that he had recently seen the "terrific" reviews of his Broadway performance. "It is certainly understandable that you, who could play a paraplegic with such honesty and realism, would be interested in and receptive to the needs of people like myself and my fellow patients here at Carville who have Hansen's disease." Stein invited Brando to visit Carville to see the facility for himself. He also mentioned the aborted movie deal with Columbia—"we thought Hollywood was coming to our rescue"— and said the plan now was to produce a sixteen-millimeter movie about the leprosarium that could be shown to interested groups, like clubs. Stein suggested that maybe Brando could narrate the project. "It would really put the film across with a bang," Stein wrote. Ever the salesman, he added this postscript to his letter: "Probably you are a busy guy, but do take time out and read *The Star*. I am enclosing a few copies. Anyway, please read the marked items."[14]

There's no record that Brando ever followed through, but Stein and the others were elated by all the attention. They hoped it might counteract what they saw as the "deafness" of the Public Health Service. Stein had concluded long ago that "this deafness . . . must be caused by the fact that our protest did not have a broad enough base to impress Washington."[15] The only solution seemed to be drumming up as much support as possible outside the hospital. The patients courted not only veterans and celebrities but also journalists. Stein called local and national reporters frequently to get the Carville story out.

The patients also created a network with thousands of other

Hansen's disease patients in leprosaria around the world, exchanging letters and sharing news about the latest medical developments. Escaped patient Willard Centlivre had warned Washington officials thirty years earlier that those afflicted with leprosy had organized a fraternity. Now it was true. Among other things, this patient network had pressured authorities to allow Filipina Joey Guerrero to come to the United States and to be admitted to Carville. By 1952, *The Star* had a circulation of 6,500 and was distributed in every state as well as in numerous other countries. The newspaper was becoming so influential that it was banned by health authorities in Brazil. "*The Star* was resented because our accounts of sulfone therapy caused discontent, bordering on revolt, among Brazilian patients still being treated with chaulmoogra oil," said Stein.[16]

————

Despite the progress made in treating patients with sulfone drugs, promin and diasone did not work for everyone, and when they did work, in many cases they worked very slowly. Some patients also experienced toxic side effects. Doctors at Carville, along with Sister Hilary, continued to search for alternatives, a little like chefs who had the basic ingredients for a fabulous dish but had yet to perfect the recipe. It was slow, tedious work. In 1948 and 1949, they tested a new sulfone drug, promacetin, on twenty-seven patients. Those taking the drug had few negative side effects and showed a noticeable improvement after only a few months of treatment. Sister Hilary tracked the experiment with detailed lab tests and photos of transformed faces and bodies. She coauthored a paper with Carville's doctors, noting that the test subjects had increased appetites and weight gain, "an air of well being" and fewer destructive bacilli present in their bodies.[17] It was still not a surefire cure. But getting discharged from Carville was becoming a reality for more patients every day, and the ones who remained were getting healthier.

Stein was among those whose condition was improving. But a year after that initial phone call with Bankhead, he had yet to accept her invitation to visit, even though he was eligible for a short medical leave. His first ten monthly tests in 1951 were all negative, which meant he needed only two more consecutive negative results to be discharged. Suddenly, Stein faced the real possibility that he would be able to leave the hospital after having been confined there for more than twenty years. But he was nervous about doing so. When some old friends from Texas stopped by unexpectedly to see him, he started to shake all over and confided in another patient that he "had stage fright" about meeting them. After the visit went well, Stein began to consider Bankhead's offer more seriously, although he was haunted by the memory of his last trip to New York, when his hotel sheets were burned and he was all but run out of town. Stein decided to wait for his eleventh skin test before deciding. He did not sleep the night before the results were due or eat breakfast that morning. When the phone rang in his office at *The Star* later that day, he waited several rings before picking it up. Sister Hilary was on the other end. "Congratulations!" she said. "It's negative."[18]

Still, Stein hesitated. Maybe he should wait for his twelfth test? How could he get around New York now that he was completely blind? Carville administrators agreed to provide an aide to travel with him. "Go now, while you have the chance," encouraged Dr. Jo. It was a once-in-a-lifetime opportunity.

Finally, Stein agreed. He boarded a train bound for New York shortly before Thanksgiving, and Hans Hornbostel was there to greet him when he arrived at Penn Station in midtown Manhattan. The major then took Stein to a nearby hotel, where Gertrude was waiting. Stein's reception could not have been more different from the one he had received during his last trip to New York. This time the hotel's publicity department had alerted the press so a couple of reporters were on hand to interview the now-famous leprosy patient.

The next day, Bankhead sent a car to bring Stein to her Westchester County home—called Windows because it had so many— for dinner. Stein was nervous about finally meeting the famous actress in person after a year of talking to her over the phone, but his butterflies quickly disappeared. "She enveloped me in her arms the moment I stepped out of the car, and from then on we hit it off beautifully," he wrote to his Carville friends.[19] Bankhead had grown up in Alabama and showered her blind guest with Southern hospitality. She had her cook prepare fried chicken "especially for you, darling, because you can handle it easily." She also invited several other guests, including actor Glenn Anders, who was her sometime lover. When Stein asked her where Anders was when he arrived, Bankhead replied, "He is upstairs reading *The Star*, darling. I wanted him to become familiar with your work before meeting you."[20]

After a hearty meal and a few rounds of scotch, Stein and another guest began singing duets. It was a "delightful party," he reported back to his Carville friends. A kind of "coming out party" for a man who had been isolated so long.

That was just the beginning. Bankhead had secured hard-to-get Broadway tickets so Stein could attend eight hit shows while he was in town, including *The King and I*, *South Pacific*, and *Guys and Dolls*. She also saved him a front-row seat in NBC's Radio City studio for a live broadcast of her popular new radio program, *The Big Show*. Afterward, he went to Bankhead's Manhattan apartment for the cast party, and a newspaper photographer took a picture of Bankhead and Stein, cocktails in hands, as they sat on her bed ("Please don't get any ideas," he wrote to his friends). They were nestled together, with Bankhead's arm lying across Stein's shoulder and his arm around her waist. Bankhead's eyes were shut as he planted a kiss above her right eye. Clearly, the famous actress had no fear of the disease, which was exactly the message Stein hoped to get out.

Stein also attended a banquet sponsored by the Forty and Eight veterans' group, where he was presented with more than one hundred new subscriptions to *The Star*. He spent Thanksgiving Day at the Hornbostels' house on Long Island, where he was met by a reporter and a photographer, whom Gertrude then invited to join them for dinner. "I'm afraid that I shall never come down to earth again," Stein wrote his friends that week, signing off, "Much love and hasta la vista."

From New York, Stein took his first-ever plane trip, to Chicago, to speak to a group of students and faculty at the University of Illinois Medical College. He was invited there by Dr. Frederick C. Lendrum, a physician who had written extensively about the origins and stigma of the word *leprosy*. Lendrum argued that "a person who is branded as a leper suffers more from the word than from the disease." Stein also visited nearby Abbott Laboratories, where the sulfone drug diasone was made.

The whirlwind two-and-a-half-week trip was an extraordinary excursion for a man who had been isolated on the same 350 acres for two decades. It also provided far more publicity for Carville than Stein could have hoped for. Nationally syndicated columnist Robert Ruark, one of those who interviewed Stein in New York, wrote that the *Star* editor poured "a superhuman effort into changing the disease from a near-criminal status into its true concept of a mildly contagious ailment, subject to arrest in old cases, cure in new cases. He has fought and yelled and hollered until a great many of the archaic approaches to leprosy have been abandoned." Ruark's column appeared in 176 newspapers across the country. He ended the article by saying that he told the cab driver who picked him up after his interview with Stein that he had just been with someone who had leprosy. Ruark then asked the cabbie if he would hesitate to accept his money. "Hesitate, hell," the driver reportedly responded. "That Hansom's disease, or whatever they call it now, ain't any more contagious than anything else. Hand me the dough, Mac."[21] A farfetched story, perhaps, but right on message.

When he was finally back at Carville—exhausted but elated—Stein wrote Bankhead that the trip "was like sitting a hungry man down to a feast." He also told her he had some good news to share. He had finally received his twelfth negative test result and "realized my dream. What you and other friends did for me, I shall now try to do for others."[22] Stein said he was "wildly happy" but also a little sad because he would be leaving his closest friends. He made arrangements for *The Star* to continue its crusade without his leadership and to sell his cottage to another patient. He called his mother to let her know he would be home after New Year's. A reporter from the *St. Louis Post-Dispatch* even flew in to write a feature story about Stein's "Victory over Hansen's Disease." Dr. Jo offered Stein his congratulations. Everything seemed on track for his discharge.[23]

Stein had forgotten that, as a patient, he was still at the mercy of others. Three weeks after his twelfth negative test, he had yet to receive the official word about his release. Finally, Dr. Jo called Stein into his office to tell him that there appeared to be a problem. The hospital's clinical director, Dr. Rolla Wolcott, had decided to require a follow-up medical-board exam before discharging Stein, something he could do at his discretion. This was extremely bad news for Stein, because the two men did not get along. Wolcott was one of those who had wanted to shut down *The Star* after Stein published the editorial supporting Gertrude Hornbostel's complaint about doctors not respecting the patients' privacy. When Stein got the word that he was not yet free to go, he was speechless. "I was furious, but my fury was frozen by an overwhelming chill of despair. All I could do was shake my head."[24]

The medical-board exam was scheduled for January 15, but when Stein entered the exam room, the only person there was Wolcott. Dr. Jo, who was also on the board, was away for a few days. Stein sat nervously as Wolcott used a razor blade to take six skin scrapings from his body to be tested for signs that the bacillus was still present. The doctor targeted the most likely places for the microbes—earlobe, right back, right chest, left thigh, and two spots on his left back. Stein returned to his cottage and waited.

After three nerve-racking days, he summoned the courage to go to Wolcott's office and ask what the doctor had seen under the microscope. Walcott told him that one of the skin specimens had revealed the presence of a small number of bacilli. Although he was unable to determine whether the bacteria were dead or alive, Wolcott concluded that Stein's condition "does not meet the criteria for the arrest of leprosy at this time." His discharge was denied.[25]

Stein was flabbergasted. For the first time in his life, he considered killing himself. He had just spent an incredible two weeks in New York and Chicago, mingling with celebrities, doctors, journalists, and other dignitaries. Now, he was being reminded in the starkest way that his life was not his own. He was still a prisoner, despite widespread recognition that the disease was not a serious threat to public health. Stein had the option of taking a "medical discharge," but this came with numerous restrictions and required his physician to regularly report to Carville about his condition. Stein refused on principle. That spring his health took a turn for the worse. His monthly skin test came back positive again, a turnaround he blamed on the stress of disappointment.

In August 1952, Stein was invited by an old friend to come speak at an American Legion convention in Dallas, and he was given permission to go. It turned out to be another heady experience for Stein. He shared the stage with Texas governor Allan Shivers and the state's U.S. senator—and future president—Lyndon Johnson. The audience greeted Stein enthusiastically, which was a big boost to his damaged morale. On the way back to Carville, he asked his driver to stop in San Antonio so he could visit his mother. "It was the first time my mother had embraced me since I had lost my sight, and I think the realization that I was blind struck her with its full force for the first time," he wrote. But for him, the trip was reinvigorating. "When I got back to Carville, I felt I was in control of myself once more."[26]

Stein was at work at *The Star* in June of 1953 when the new chief medical officer arrived and made the rounds. Dr. Edward "Eddie" Gordon had been hired to replace Dr. Jo, who, much to the patients' chagrin, had reached mandatory retirement age. Dr. Jo had been a strong defender of the patients, and everyone hoped that Gordon would continue that relationship. The patients knew they were vulnerable to the impulses of each new medical director, so they were encouraged when Gordon showed up with a slightly goofy grin and, as one resident put it, "pleasant smiling" eyes. He also had what Stein called "an incipient double chin." The sisters described the new director as "very quiet and unassuming."[27] He seemed harmless enough.

It didn't take long before the patients realized how wrong they were. The forty-eight-year-old Gordon had spent his entire career in the Public Health Service and was a hospital administrator to the core. He liked to run a tight ship. Some of his initial decisions were popular. He shut down the Carville jail and hired trained attendants to replace the patients who worked as orderlies but were often ill-equipped to do the job.

Then Gordon issued a directive that left Carville and its 350 residents reeling. He ordered all able-bodied individuals with arrested cases of the disease to leave. Those with disabilities were "invited" to leave. It was a stunning—almost unthinkable—turnaround for people who had been institutionalized against their will for so many years. It was one thing to be allowed to go. It was another to be forced to do so. Some patients had been confined for so long they'd grown dependent on Carville and had nowhere else to go. They had no work skills or experience and feared they would be unable to survive on their own. Suddenly their worlds had flipped.

The patients called for an emergency meeting with Gordon and Wolcott, who was still clinical director. They pointed out that some residents no longer had families or friends outside to support them. Others had crippled hands and feet, and would be ostracized once people found out where they had been. The patients argued that the government had upended their lives by forcing them to come to the leprosy hospital in the first place. It couldn't just toss them out. The patients suggested a compromise, that the order apply only to those who had been at Carville for less than three years.[28]

Gordon would not budge. "We do not consider our hospitalization charity," he responded curtly.[29] Eligible patients were told they had three months to move out. Gordon argued that reintegrating patients back into society was part of educating the public that people who had Hansen's disease were able to resume a normal life and should not be feared. The patients agreed that such education was crucial, but objected that they were the ones being forced to do the teaching.

To Gordon, Carville was a hospital where people came to be treated for a disease. For patients, it was both a hospital and a home, the place where they tried to piece together lives that had been disrupted through no fault of their own. It was a place where some of them had spent almost their entire lives, making friends, going to school, falling in love, and growing old. But some health officials in Washington believed that the patients were taking advantage of the government and were not appreciative enough of the free care they received. The new medical officer in charge had clearly been sent there to clean house.

To keep up the pressure, Gordon declared that patients with arrested cases could no longer hold jobs at the facility, or even at patient-run operations such as the canteen or the shops they had set up to provide services such as bike repairs. He ordered that only one spouse at a time could hold a job at the leprosarium, a big blow to couples who were trying to save enough money to live on their own if and when they were discharged. He also said that discharged patients could no longer sell their cottages to other patients, and that the buildings—which the patients had built and paid for with their own money—were now the property of the U.S. government. Gordon had bulldozers knock down some of the more unsightly structures, including patients' chicken coops and rabbit hutches. They were no longer allowed to raise animals. He was taking away everything that had given the patients some sense of independence and normalcy.[30]

Among those who had to leave Carville that year was Johnny Harmon. He was able to move nearby to be close to his two children and to set up a photography business, but he had to leave his wife behind. "I will never forget how lonely I felt as I drove down the winding river road to Vacherie with a 4x5 photographic enlarger at my side where my wife usually rode."[31]

Gordon made other changes that reduced Carville's contact with the outside world. Visiting hours were cut back, a big setback for the patients' campaign to enlighten the public by opening up the grounds to anyone who wanted to see the leprosarium. Gordon also had the notorious "hole in the fence" sealed up. *The Star* noted that twenty-three patients absconded from Carville during the new director's first full year on the job. "They were probably seeking a change impossible to bring about here—change of climate," the paper said.

Gordon especially upset patients when he ordered the immediate removal of more than a dozen patients who had come to Carville four years earlier from the U.S. Virgin Islands. Dr. Jo, at the urging of *The Star*, had admitted them because conditions at their hospital in St. Croix were extremely poor and the patients were deprived of the latest medical treatment, including reconstructive surgery on hands and feet. The Virgin Islanders' arrival in 1951 had been big news at Carville and a large crowd of patients gathered at the infirmary to greet them. "It had the appearance of a catastrophe to see them enter, some carried in on stretchers, some brought in on wheelchairs and among them many blind—the blind, the maimed, the incapacitated," the Daughters of Charity wrote in their annals.[32]

Among the arrivals was twenty-three-year-old Simeon Peterson, who had been confined at the St. Croix hospital since the age of six. For him, Carville was a dream come true. In the Virgin Islands, "you went to the hospital and you stay there until you die," he said. "Nobody want you. People scared. Your family won't receive you." Peterson's mother was the only person who ever visited him, and she came only once a month. When she did, she was not allowed to touch her son. Peterson discovered a whole new life at Carville, a place where he could make lots of friends and there were plenty of activities to keep a young man occupied. Doctors were also able to operate on his crippled hands, replacing tendons immobilized by Hansen's disease, so he could use his hands again. At Carville, Peterson was allowed to thrive.[33]

But in 1955, Gordon declared that the Virgin Island patients had received all the extra care they needed. They were given three days to pack up and return to the islands. "It struck us like an atomic attack, suddenly and without warning," said one of the patients.[34] Seven of them immediately ran away. It was rumored that they headed north, where they were less likely to be found. Publicly, Gordon downplayed the escape, assuring the public that there was little to worry about. "We don't like them to leave without our knowledge, but there is no federal law that I know of which was violated," he said, a reference to the fact that it was still up to state health authorities, not the federal government, to order that patients be confined.

The seven other Virgin Islanders were taken a couple of days later to the Baton Rouge airport and put on a plane for St. Croix. Six of them had arrested cases of the disease and carried letters that they hoped would keep them from being readmitted to the old leprosy hospital, where they knew conditions remained deplorable. The St. Croix facility was an eight-acre site surrounded by a high wire fence, located next to a vile-smelling rum distillery. The buildings had dirt floors and no baths and were infested with rats. One visitor called the hospital "a disgrace to the American flag." The patients were distraught to have to go back after all these years, and it's not clear what ultimately became of them. Peterson, known fondly at Carville as Mr. Pete, was among the few Virgin Islanders allowed to stay in Louisiana.

By the summer of 1956, tensions between Gordon and the hospital's remaining 310 patients had reached the boiling point. They were upset by his decision to raise the minimum visiting age for nonrelatives from sixteen to twenty. But they were outraged when he banned outsiders from participating in patient activities, such as softball games, golf tournaments, and dances. The patients were also told that they could no longer dance with nonpatients at dances held in the recreation center, even if they were married.

Such community activities had been sanctioned, even encouraged, in the past and were among the most anticipated events of the year. They made the patients feel almost like normal human beings. Playing sports against outsiders especially gave them confidence that they might someday be able to function in the world beyond Carville. "To be able to compete with a well person and win did a patient almost as much good as all the medicine in the world," wrote Baton Rouge *State-Times* sportswriter Bill Williams.[35] When the Carville Indians had won the River League softball championship in 1951, competing against teams from Baton Rouge and nearby, the entire hospital erupted in celebration. The patients were also proud of their team's diversity. The players included four Mexican Americans, three blacks, one Hawaiian, one Samoan, three Japanese Americans, and four whites.[36] Their star pitcher was black—seventeen-year-old Richard Williams, who had been a patient at Carville since the age of six and drew glowing attention from the local press. Now Gordon wanted it to end.

The director insisted that he was merely trying to protect the public. "In deference to the fact that leprosy is a communicable disease and in consideration of the health of others, patients should have as few and as casual contacts with non-patients as possible," he said.[37] Gordon had adopted the minority view at the Public Health Service that Hansen's disease was more contagious than most medical experts believed. At least he wanted to err on the side of caution. When asked by a reporter about his order blocking outside participation in Carville events and raising the minimum age for visitors, Gordon replied, "I wouldn't let my kids do it. Why should I let yours?"[38]

The new restrictions seemed not only unnecessary but cruel. Everything the patients had struggled so hard to achieve was being taken away. Besides fighting for the right to leave, they now had to fight for the right to stay. There were rumors that *The Star*—which now had up to ten thousand subscribers—was under threat of being shut down.[39] It also appeared that the patients' cherished Cottage Grove might be slated for demolition. The patients knew they had to get a lot more aggressive. This was war.

Chapter 17

Human Touch

THE FIRST THING the patients did was to go on strike. If they were not allowed to hold social events with nonpatients—activities they craved—they wouldn't hold them at all. A dance scheduled for the high school graduation that summer was canceled, as was the Halloween dance in the fall and a much-anticipated Veterans' Day program. The patients knew this would not look good for the Public Health Service.

The second thing they did was to hire a lawyer, Robert L. Kleinpeter of Baton Rouge. The son of a legionnaire, Kleinpeter had accompanied his father to Carville as a boy and performed tap dances for the patients. Now, he was going to Washington to lobby on their behalf. Kleinpeter brought with him a scathing five-page letter from the Patients' Federation, which called on the surgeon general to replace the much despised chief medical officer. "We regret that the doctor-patient relationship has deteriorated to the point where it has become intolerable," the patients wrote. They said they no longer had respect for and confidence in Gordon, who "does not seem to have the human touch."[1]

The patients noted that anger at the hospital was so intense, someone had chalked "insulting" words about Gordon along the screened-in walkways of the compound. A Public Health Service sign had also been defaced, with the "USPHS" crossed out and "USSR" written underneath, at a time when being linked to Communist Russia was no joke. "While we deplore such action, one must bear in mind that there are a number of patients here at Carville who have no other way of venting their feelings," the federation wrote to the surgeon general, adding that patients feared that if they opposed Gordon too openly "they may be singled out for personal retaliation." Some patients were especially nervous about losing their part-time jobs. Such jobs, noted one resident, gave them "something to do" and kept them "from going nuts."

Kleinpeter reported back to his clients that he was making progress and believed many of their concerns would be addressed. But the patients were unwilling to leave anything to chance. They were also reluctant to rely on *The Star* to take the lead in the dispute, because Gordon and others in the Public Health Service seemed eager to find any excuse to shut the newspaper down. So patients took their story to the local newspapers. "Carville Patients Protest New Rules by Medical Director," reported the Baton Rouge *Morning Advocate* on August 5, 1956. "Clamp-Down at Carville Is Protested," read the *Shreveport Times*. Gordon was quoted in the articles saying that he was only trying to protect public health. The medical officer admitted that he had heard rumors of the patients' complaints, but insisted that he had not been personally approached by any of the patients.

It was an implausible claim, given the raucous three-hour confrontation he'd had with them a few days earlier. Gordon and top

public health authorities from Washington had called a meeting in
the theater of the recreation building to discuss the future of Cottage Grove. For several years, they had been concerned about the
safety of the haphazardly built structures and were eager to tear
them down. The time had come. Half a dozen officials sat behind a
long metal table in front of the stage. Stein and other cottage residents sat facing them in the theater seats. Dr. C. K. Himmelsbach,
head of the Public Health Service's hospital division, opened the
meeting by announcing that the government planned to tear all
eighteen cottages down. The residents would have to move back
into the dorms, although some of those would be remodeled to provide apartments for married couples. Each apartment would have
a living room, bedroom, and bath, but no kitchen, which meant an
end to home-cooked meals; everyone would now have to eat in the
cafeteria.[2]

The patients were stunned. This was the last straw. These little cottages, as rickety as they might have appeared, were their
homes. They were the only places where patients enjoyed some
semblance of freedom. The residents entertained their friends
there, raised pets, tended gardens, and prepared the kinds of food
they had grown up with—whether it was Mexican, Chinese, Italian, or Cajun. Having a place they could call their own eased some
of the intense pain of being removed from family and friends. "It's
like being emancipated back there," one resident told the officials.
The patients knew that Congress had recently approved $25,000
for the government to buy the cottages, but they had been led to
believe that the structures would be fixed up and reassigned. Himmelsbach said they were mistaken. They would have to give up not
only their houses but also their furniture and, most disturbingly to
some, their pets, which were not allowed in the dorms.

Himmelsbach and Gordon were taken aback by the patients'
reaction and seemed to have no idea why they were so upset. Gor-

don said he was especially surprised that the women in the audience did not welcome having someone else do the cooking. "I do not know what prevents you from eating in the dining room," he told them. Himmelsbach also insisted that doctors needed to know what their patients were eating, which was not possible when patients prepared their own meals. "Food is an important part in the therapy of this disease, and I want the diet supervised," he said. Himmelsbach added that the patients were only being asked to do what many couples around the country did, which was to live in an apartment. To which one patient replied that those people were free to come and go as they pleased, and to choose for themselves whether they ate at home or in a restaurant. "If you have a chance to live in a home or a hotel room, in which would you live?" a patient asked.

The divide in the room was as wide and deep as the river outside, and it seemed to grow wider as the debate dragged on. The patients believed that Gordon and the others were missing the point. Carville was not a normal hospital where people stayed for a few days or weeks, but an institution where they lived for years or even decades. Many patients stayed—rather than escape through the hole in the fence—only because they believed what they had been told, that their isolation was beneficial to public health. That didn't mean they couldn't make the best of it. "Is this a hospital or a hospital community?" one man called out. To which Gordon bluntly replied, "A hospital." The medical officer became so frustrated at one point that he rose from his chair and pounded the table, shouting that married patients "for some strange reason" felt entitled to having their own cottages. "Is it not a fact that sometimes we have to be satisfied with something that is a little less than ideal?" he demanded. The patients were unmoved. These were their homes. At its core, the dispute was about control, and Gordon wanted to show that he was in charge. "When you are running a railroad there are certain rules to go by. Running a hospital is the same way," he told the patients. The plan would go forward.

The patients were not so easily silenced. They decided to recruit their friends in the American Legion and other veterans' groups to pass resolutions calling on the Public Health Service to reconsider the plan. They portrayed it as a fight for their health and well-being, in an appeal for public sympathy. Ann Autry, president of the Baton Rouge Ladies Auxiliary of the Veterans of Foreign Wars, called on her members to lobby on the patients' behalf. "I know that our congressman did not intend to set the progress of treatment of Hansen's disease back 50 years," she told them.[3]

It was a public spat that the health service had hoped to avoid, but it could hardly have been a surprise. Internal Public Health Service documents noted a few years earlier that taking the cottages away from the patients would be "a very delicate situation. It has tremendous public relations aspects." And indeed it did.[4]

On August 23, Congressman Otto Passman, from Monroe, Louisiana, flew down from Washington to find out what all the ruckus was about. Carville patients were harder for politicians to ignore now that they had become an active voting bloc. The conservative Democrat was a member of the House Appropriations Committee, the panel that had approved the funds to buy the patients' cottages. When Passman arrived at Gordon's office, he found a reporter from the Baton Rouge *State-Times* interviewing the director for a five-part series about the unrest at Carville. It was not a good sign. Gordon insisted to both the reporter and the congressman that his demands were reasonable. The cottages were old and unsafe, he said, and the patients would be better cared for in the dorms. Gordon also defended his decision to restrict the patients' access to outsiders, arguing that it was still unclear how leprosy was spread. He insisted that the patients had lots of other activities to keep them busy. "You can never please them all," he told Passman. Still, perhaps sensing he was losing the argument, Gordon agreed to the congressman's request to hold off demolishing the cottages while he looked for funding to build new ones.[5]

Passman left Gordon's office to go outside and meet with the patients. They gathered together for a box lunch on the shores of Lake Johansen, an artificial lake that had been built at the rear of the hospital grounds for drainage and recreation. It was named after the well-liked previous medical director, Dr. Jo—a fitting place to discuss the fate of his successor. "It was a pretty hot day, but the air at the Lake was brisk, and so was the discussion—brisk, detailed and, as we later came to know, ever so fruitful," *The Star* reported. Passman assured the patients that he was on their side. "Let them tear down the cottages," he said. "I'll get Congress to appropriate the money to build new and modern ones. We spend millions building hospitals all over the world; it's time we paid some attention to our own." Passman hinted that he also might call for a congressional investigation of the hospital's administration.[6]

The patients were ecstatic. This was the first time in the history of Carville that a member of Congress had come to visit. The congressman even followed up with a thank-you note, in which he called Carville residents "my fellow Americans who are presently patients there," and said that he felt "a bit ashamed of myself that I have waited so long to visit with you wonderful people." Passman oversaw U.S. foreign-aid spending and said he was not happy about all the money the United States was sending overseas. "You are citizens of this country, taxpayers and voters, and you should have more consideration from our government than foreign countries are receiving," he wrote.[7]

Local newspapers soon weighed in, portraying the Public Health Service as the clear villain in the dispute. The *Monroe Morning World* published an editorial three days after Passman's visit that was headlined "Soviet-Type Prison Camp at Carville?" The paper accused Gordon of trying to implement "a scheme to regiment the Carville patients along the lines of Soviet disciplinary barracks" and called for him to be fired. "In the meantime, all moves aimed at a Soviet-style integration of the Carville patients, into what would amount to a concentration camp, should be halted overnight," the paper said.[8] These were unusually strong words, especially so soon after World War II, but other newspapers went on to repeat them. By September, the national press was starting to take note. *Time* magazine ran an article citing Gordon's seemingly cold-hearted order prohibiting patients from dancing with nonpatients, even if they were their spouses. Louisiana congressman Hale Boggs called for an investigation.[9]

Gordon's supporters tried desperately to save his job. Carville employees still received hazard pay and some of them thought Gordon's departure would enable the patients to push for changes that might endanger their extra wages, or even their jobs. On September 10, the American Legion post in nearby St. Gabriel, whose members included many hospital employees, approved a resolution calling the criticism of Gordon unjustified. The resolution, which was directed at the surgeon general, noted that leprosy remained a quarantinable disease in Louisiana and urged the Public Health Service to "take a firm stand on visiting privileges, etc., in the interest of safeguarding public health."[10] *The Star* reported that this same group of employees, including two department heads, had circulated a petition earlier among hospital personnel calling for Gordon to be retained. "Do you want the patients to run the hospital instead of the doctors? If they win out, there's no stopping them," the staffers had told their fellow employees, according to *The Star*.[11]

For Gordon, it was too late. On September 13, Passman released a statement to the press announcing that the medical director was out. He was to be transferred and replaced by another Public

Health Service doctor, Edgar B. Johnwick, a forty-eight-year-old skin specialist. The assistant surgeon general, Jack Masur, flew down from Washington that same day to do some quick damage control. He told the patients that Gordon was being transferred at his own request, something few believed. Masur also condemned the *Time* magazine article, calling it "unfortunate for all of us. It smacks of yellow journalism." He added, "I am asking all people concerned to lay hands off and quiet things down." The patients were happy to oblige, now that they had what they wanted. The head of the Patients' Federation, Darryl Broussard, announced that the canceled social events were back on.

———

The contrast between Gordon and Johnwick could not have been greater. The new director arrived at Carville shortly before Thanksgiving 1956, and within days the patients knew things had changed. One of Johnwick's first acts was to call the entire staff, medical personnel, and patients together, something that had never been done before. Several hundred people gathered in the same theater where, less than three months earlier, Gordon and Himmelsbach had confronted the patients over the fate of Cottage Grove. Speaking to the anxious crowd, Johnwick told them that they all had to work together. They were a team. He said Carville had three missions: providing the best medical care, conducting research to help millions of leprosy patients around the world, and sharing knowledge about the disease. "These three things are not done separately by different members of the staff but by a team that is made up of the staff and patients. It is my privilege to be the captain of this team and it is my duty to help this team accomplish its missions," he told the crowd.[12]

The new director then made an astounding declaration. "No one should be discharged from this hospital against his will. No one should be kept in this hospital against his will." This was everything the patients had hoped for. It would still be a few more years before the last American with Hansen's disease was forced to go to Carville—and disputes over forced discharges would continue for decades—but Johnwick's statement was revolutionary. "The tension which hung over this hospital like a heavy fog, had lifted," reported *The Star*. "There was a sudden and profound change in climate."

The new medical director further endeared himself to the patients by rereading his speech in Spanish for the benefit of the many Spanish-speaking residents. He also promised to be available every afternoon in the infirmary to meet with patients. "Patients' morale is zooming," said *The Star*. The paper noted that a golf tournament banned by Gordon had been rescheduled and was expected to attract about fifty golfers from Baton Rouge, New Orleans, and other surrounding towns. Johnwick said the tournament was good for community relations and for patients' morale, which was also good for their health.[13] A few days after his speech, Johnwick visited the Cottage Grove residents to talk about their future. He told them that the government would replace their existing cottages with new, modern ones and that married couples who moved to the dorms would have their own kitchens. "Happy Days are here again!" proclaimed *The Star*.

––––––

The outside world was not quite as encouraging. The flurry of postwar publicity, spurred by Tallulah Bankhead, the Hornbostels, Joey Guerrero, and others, had faded away by the late 1950s. The nation had more pressing concerns. There was an intense worldwide campaign to eradicate polio, which paralyzed thousands of Americans each year. Cold War fears that the Soviet Union might drop a nuclear bomb on the United States had schoolchildren scuttling under their desks. The fight to secure civil rights for black Americans easily overshadowed the discrimination faced by a few hundred leprosy patients.

Betty and Harry Martin knew better than most the challenges the patients faced. As ecstatic as they had been to be out on their own, they were struggling to build a new life for themselves outside Carville. They craved a fresh start, so they moved away from Louisiana, first to North Carolina and then to California, as far as they could get from their past. But Harry found it almost impossible to find work. He had no references or experience and did not want to reveal where he had been for the last twenty years of his life. That made potential employers suspicious and he found one door after another shut in his face. He could find only low-paying and physically demanding jobs, selling household supplies door to door in North Carolina and driving a truck in California. The Martins, now in their early forties, realized that they were ill-equipped to handle themselves in the outside world. They had a hard time making new friends and were frequently cheated by unscrupulous salesmen. "We were beginning to realize that our many years inside the hospital had weakened our capacity for independence," wrote Betty.[14]

The Martins also lived in constant fear that their past would be exposed and they would be ostracized by those around them. So they mostly kept to themselves, almost like criminals on the lam. "We are always afraid," said Betty, who worried that any day they might have to pick up and flee. It drove them to despair. Betty wrote a second book, called *No One Must Ever Know*, which came out in 1959, again using her Carville alias. The Martins had finally achieved one of their dreams, buying a small house on a hill in California but, wrote Betty, "The truth is that our fear of the stigma has grown instead of lessened because we now have more to lose if we are exposed."[15]

Some at Carville bristled at the Martins' excessive fear of having their identities revealed. These patients and staffers believed that times were changing and that discharged patients could resume normal lives. Indeed, some of the younger patients who had left the hospital found that to be the case, including a Texan named Julia Elwood, who made no secret of her background and was able to find an office job in Baton Rouge. She later became the first former patient hired as a regular employee at Carville.[16] Some of the patients argued that they would never be accepted in society if those among them continued to hide the truth. In reviewing Betty Martin's book, one medical expert said it would have been more helpful if the author had called it *Everyone Must Know.*[17]

Betty recognized that their anxiety was preventing them from getting better, and the couple found themselves returning to Carville periodically for medical care. Harry needed reconstructive surgery on his hands, which had been crippled by the bacilli and further damaged by the manual jobs he took to pay the bills. Betty's disease had also reappeared, although it was still an extremely mild case. At least at Carville, they knew they would be surrounded by people who understood and cared about them. Medical services had greatly improved since their departure more than a decade before, with more physical therapy, rehabilitation, and plastic surgery to help patients prepare for the outside world. "Carville was now a great modern hospital in every sense of the word," wrote Betty.[18]

Still, it was largely left up to the patients and their advocates to cure public misperceptions. Many people remained suspicious of and repelled by the disease, and the government was doing little to change their minds. The tireless Stanley Stein continued his campaign, monitoring publications and broadcasts for misleading information so he could dash off letters demanding corrections. Ludwig Lederer, who wrote a science column in the

Hartford Courant, was the recipient of one of Stein's many missives. Lederer had written about a thirty-five-year-old navy veteran in North Carolina who had been diagnosed with Hansen's disease. The man was eventually sent to Carville, but not before local newspapers revealed his name and his wife's teaching job was put in jeopardy. "Stanley Stein, the editor of *The Star*, points out that the publicity given to the leprosy case in North Carolina created a panic in parts of the state and had most unpleasant consequences for the family of the unfortunate patient," wrote a repentant Lederer. He then went on to correct some common myths about Hansen's disease, informing readers that leprosy was difficult to contract and that the modern illness was not the same as the one depicted in the Bible.[19]

Popular columnist Ann Landers also addressed the issue after two schoolchildren wrote to tell her that their teacher said Landers was incorrect when she claimed that leprosy was one of the least contagious diseases. "The teacher says she hopes you will be big enough to print this letter and admit your mistake because you are giving people the wrong impression," the children wrote. Landers replied in her column that it was their teacher who was mistaken, because "all medical authorities who have studied leprosy (Hansen's disease) agree that it is not easily transmitted." Landers noted that not one worker at the Carville leprosarium had contracted the disease in over sixty years. She ended by saying that she hoped the girls' teacher would read Lander's column in class "because she is giving people the wrong impression."[20]

These were minor victories, to be sure, in the battle to reverse a centuries-old stigma. The myths about leprosy were clearly baked into the public psyche, and people still instinctively recoiled at the mere mention of the disease. Even those who knew better were reluctant to take chances. When Tom Kelly, a reporter for the *New Orleans Item*, was engaged to be married in the early 1950s, he brought his fiancée, Marguerite Lelong, to Carville to meet his aunt, Sister Teresa Kelly, who was the head nurse at the time. Marguerite said Sister Teresa took her into her office and they went through the files together to make certain she was not related to any of the patients and potentially vulnerable to the disease. Marguerite was cleared and she and Tom got married. On another occasion, Tom took one of his newspaper colleagues to Carville to meet Stanley Stein, by then a local celebrity. But when the colleague got up to leave the meeting, he froze at the door. He couldn't get himself to touch the knob. After an uncomfortable silence, someone else in the room finally got up and opened the door.[21]

————

It took almost three years, but finally the Cottage Grove homes were set to come down. On the morning of May 25, 1959, a bulldozer began razing the eighteen small houses, grinding up years of memories along with pieces of wood, windows, and discarded furniture. *The Star* reported that the workmen then "set fire to a pile of rubble and in so doing brought to a flaming close an era of Carville's erratic history." Many Cottage Grove occupants had lived in their houses longer than the average American family. As the wooden structures turned into ash, other workmen were busy building ten modern brick houses nearby, where some of the married couples would eventually live. One of the dorms was also being renovated to make twelve new apartments. Cottage Grove would never be the same.[22]

Stanley Stein was one of those who would have to move back to the dorms. Because he was not married, he was not eligible for one of the new homes. Stein had lived in his cottage, Wits' End, for twenty-five years. It had become a central gathering place for patients and visitors, and was the base from which the insurgent campaign against Gordon had been launched. Stein said one of the advantages of being blind as the demolition began was that "I could not see the heartbreaking spectacle of the equally blind machines running rough-shod over nearly half my life."[23] The disadvantage was that he would now have to learn his way around an unfamiliar dorm room, touching walls and furniture he was unable to see.

Stein would also lose his best friend, a twelve-year-old black-and-white Boston terrier named Bing. The two had been inseparable since the dog was only five weeks old. Stein could not bring him to the dorm, so Bing was taken to a kennel at the back of the hospital grounds to live. But the first night in his new home Bing howled and barked incessantly. On the second night he escaped and was found frantically running around Stein's empty cottage, barking, looking for his owner. A passing patient picked him up and snuck the dog into Stein's dorm room to spend the night, but Bing was later returned to the kennel and died less than two months later. "I think change hastened his death," said Stein. The dog was buried under a magnolia tree on what used to be the front yard of Wits' End.[24]

Chapter 18

An Era Ends

STEIN AND THE other patients had had high expectations, with so many promising developments in medical research. They were certain that sulfones would finally end their exile. Instead, as the rest of the nation throbbed with postwar optimism, Carville residents found themselves once again forgotten and left behind. Sulfone drugs arrested a large number of cases, but they did not work for everyone, and no one knew why.

More than a hundred years after Norway's Dr. Danielssen had failed to inoculate himself with *Mycobacterium leprae*, researchers were still unable to grow the Hansen's bacilli outside the human body in a meaningful way. One Public Health Service doctor, Charles Shepard, had cultivated the germs in the footpads of mice, but those bacilli were of limited use because the mice never developed full-blown cases of leprosy. The medical community still did not know how the disease infiltrated the body, how it was spread, or how it could be stopped. There was no easy way to test whether

someone had the disease, and there was no vaccine to prevent people from getting it in the first place.

So it was with great anticipation that patients and staff greeted
a tiny French nun when she visited Carville in 1954. Sister Marie
Suzanne was a Marist Missionary who in her dark veil and habit
looked nondescript, except for a white pleated ruffle that encir-
cled her face like a piece of boxed candy. Sister Marie Suzanne
was a well-known researcher who had studied Hansen's disease
for decades, including at the prestigious Pasteur Institute in Paris.
A few years earlier, she had discovered an organism similar to
Mycobacterium leprae while examining some leprous tissue. She was
able to grow the bacteria in the lab and inject it into mice, producing lesions similar to those seen in Hansen's disease. Sister Marie
Suzanne believed that this newly discovered bacillus could be used
to develop a vaccine that would prevent someone from contracting
the disease by triggering the body's immune system. She thought
it could also be used as an antigen to ease the symptoms of those
who were already infected.[1] If true, this would be a major step forward in the effort to combat leprosy. The newly discovered bacillus
was named *Mycobacterium marianum*, in honor of the Virgin Mary,
to whom the sister had dedicated her work. She even placed a vial
of the bacilli at the foot of the hallowed statue of Our Lady of the
Grotto in Lourdes, a popular pilgrimage site in France. Faith in
God was still considered an essential ingredient for ridding the
world of leprosy.[2]

Sister Marie Suzanne came to Carville as part of a thirty-four-
city tour of the United States to discuss her work and her plans
to expand testing of her vaccine and antigen. Trials had already
begun in West Africa, with some positive outcomes. A majority
of those taking the antigen reportedly had seen their conditions
improve, and researchers were eager for more extensive results.

The sister claimed not that she had found a cure for leprosy but that she might be on to "something big." Now Sister Marie Suzanne wanted Carville patients to join in the testing.

Carville patients, as always, were eager to participate in anything they thought might improve their lives. About sixty patients agreed to take monthly injections of the *Marianum* antigen over the next two years, but in 1957, before the results were in, Sister Marie Suzanne died from a brain tumor. She was praised around the world for her work and commitment to fighting a disease that had plagued so many. A newspaper reported that one of her last requests before heading into surgery was "Don't give up the laboratory." The press played up the fact that within an hour of her death, Vatican scientists issued a report concluding that Sister Marie Suzanne had "succeeded where the medical profession had failed: She produced vaccines and related preparations which are highly effective in both the treatment and prevention of leprosy."[3] Some newspapers went further. "French Nun-Scientist Dies, Discovered Leprosy Cure," read the *Catholic Courier Journal*.

The problem was, it wasn't true. She had not discovered a cure. Neither the antigen nor the vaccine, after lengthy testing, appeared to have much effect. Dr. Johnwick reported shortly after Sister Marie Suzanne's death that while Carville patients taking the injections were still under observation, "the *Marianum* antigen has been generally ineffective here, and we cannot recommend it for general use on the basis of our experience." One of the patients trying the test drug was Stanley Stein. "In my role of perennial guinea pig, I took the shots but got no benefit from them," he reported.[4] It was another false hope.

Still, each discovery, even if unsuccessful, was seen at Carville as another step toward unlocking the secrets of leprosy. Millions of people around the world continued to suffer from the disease, and Carville was in a good position to help. A new research director, pathologist George Fite, hoped to finally turn the leprosarium into a world-class research facility. He envisioned a state-of-the-art lab with a staff of eighteen, including a bacteriologist and a chemist. Fite tried to smooth the transition before his arrival in 1959 by writing to Sister Hilary, the lab's current biochemist, to solicit her opinion about the changes he planned to make.[5]

The effort did not go well. Sister Hilary, who had spent decades in the lab, conducting countless tests and coauthoring forty-three scientific papers, was not about to let herself be pushed aside. After eight months on the job, Fite complained to Dr. Johnwick that Sister Hilary was "not humble" and had told visitors that she was not being treated fairly under the new regime. "There is not room for two 'masters' in the Laboratory Branch," wrote Fite. He said Sister Hilary needed to retire. "It is my firm and studied opinion that her future does not lie here." Sister Hilary countered by complaining to Johnwick that Fite did not want her in the lab and had assigned other people to do her work. It was not a tenable situation.[6]

In 1960, after thirty-seven years at Carville, Sister Hilary announced her retirement. At the time, she was the longest-serving Daughter of Charity at the leprosarium. Few people were aware that she was being pushed aside. Sister Hilary was sixty-six years old and no one questioned why she would leave after so many years. Instead, she was applauded for her decision to move to Japan to help the Daughters of Charity set up a new Rehabilitation Center for Crippled Children. She was showered with praise from patients, hospital staffers, and the Public Health Service for her work both inside and outside the lab. At a ceremony marking her departure, one speaker said that Sister Hilary was never one to believe that "all ye who enter here leave all hope behind." Instead, he said, "She determined that what could be blocked from the outside, could be unlocked from the inside."[7]

Besides her other jobs, Sister Hilary had been the unofficial

historian of Carville and had compiled a thick volume of photos, documents, and anecdotes covering more than sixty years.
Much of what the world would know about Carville was due to
Sister Hilary's efforts to preserve its history and her sensitivity
to both its tragedy and promise. On page 147 of her compilation
is a typical entry, an undated black-and-white photo of a young
boy dressed up as Uncle Sam for a July Fourth celebration. The
small patient is wearing striped pants, a little jacket with tails,
and a striped stovepipe hat that all but conceals his head. The boy
appears to be about six or seven years old. The caption beneath
the photo simply states that he "died at the age of 12 years." These
were the patients Sister Hilary and others at Carville had worked
so hard to heal. But now times were changing—probably for the
better. Sister Hilary noted before her departure, in her scientific,
matter-of-fact manner, that the lab in the infirmary had just been
remodeled, with stainless-steel furniture and modern equipment,
a far cry from the makeshift lab in the small cottage that she had
used when she first arrived.

As Sister Hilary was walking out the door, doctors and
researchers from around the world were walking in, some to visit
and learn about the latest work being done at Carville, others to
stay and contribute to the research. Despite its remote location,
the U.S. leprosarium had become an essential destination for those
working on Hansen's disease. "We used to say we were so deep in
the sticks we had to pipe sunshine in," said James Carville, the
prominent Democratic strategist and grandson of Louis Carville,
the town's original postmaster. But he also recalled that residents
of the tiny town were proud of the hospital and frequently boasted
that they had more doctors per capita than Rochester, Minnesota,
home of the famous Mayo Clinic. "There were a lot of educated
people there, interesting, fascinating people," he said.[8] Isadore
Dyer would have been pleased.

The fifty-five scientists who participated in a seminar at Carville in April 1965 were typical—medical professionals from countries around the world, including Liberia, Bolivia, and Vietnam. Among them was Paul Brand, a British orthopedic surgeon who had done groundbreaking work with leprosy patients in India.[9] Brand was among the first in the medical community to realize that the loss of fingers, toes, and limbs, which disabled so many Hansen's disease patients, was due more to injuries resulting from their inability to feel pain than to the body's gradual absorption of bones as a result of the disease. He reached this conclusion after watching leprosy patients in India walking around unaware that they had pieces of glass or nails stuck in their feet, because they were numb. Their untreated injuries often led to serious infections and to amputations.

Brand encouraged patients and their caregivers to take special precautions to avoid such injuries before they turned into permanent disabilities. He helped develop special footwear that allowed patients to keep their weight off sore spots, giving lesions time to heal. He also pioneered special reconstructive surgery to fix crippled hands, replacing nonfunctioning tendons with healthy ones, so patients could once again perform complex manual tasks, such as typing, sewing, and playing musical instruments.

After Brand spoke at the Carville seminar about his work, Dr. Johnwick pulled him aside and asked if he would consider joining his staff. "It's quite apparent that your patients in India get a better rehabilitation program than our patients in the United States," Johnwick said. "As an officer of the U.S. Public Health Service, I can't accept that." Within a year, Brand had moved to Carville, along with his wife—who was also a doctor and became the hospital's ophthalmologist[10]—and five of their six children. Brand found a lot to like about the place. He loved the flat, open fields covered in goldenrod and the rows of massive moss-draped oaks.

There was a lake stocked with fish, as well as a golf course, base-ball fields, government-funded entertainment, and air-conditioned buildings. The lab was modern and well equipped. "My patients' comfort level in this plantation setting far exceeded anything I had known in India," he wrote. "But leprosy finds a way to work its peculiar pattern of destruction regardless of the setting."[11]

Brand was shocked to discover that his patients faced more dis-crimination and isolation in the United States than in Asia, where the disease was more common and therefore a more accepted part of life. He was surprised that Carville patients were not allowed to visit the homes of staff members and that children under the age of sixteen, including his own, were forbidden from going to the patient side of the complex. Brand called the sterilization of the patients' mail before it left the grounds "an absurd and medically useless practice."

His children, who had been raised in India, were as disturbed as he was. One of his daughters balked at getting married in the Carville mansion because none of the patients were allowed to attend. His youngest daughter would tease Americans about their leprophobia, by running to the fence, curling up her fingers, and making a scrunched-up face whenever she saw a car slow down outside, so the passengers could catch sight of a "leper." The Brands also found it hard to believe that some patients had been brought to the hospital in chains and that most were encouraged to change their names to protect their families from shame.

Paul Brand, whose gentle manner and warm smile earned him the nickname St. Paul, learned much about the history of Car-ville from a patient he already knew by reputation. Stanley Stein was an international figure by this time, famous among Hansen's disease workers and victims for his efforts to confront public prej-udice. He had recently written his own book, called *Alone No Lon-ger: The Story of a Man Who Refused to Be One of the Living Dead*. Now in his sixties, Stein still edited *The Star* and continued to crusade against use of the word *leper* and to correct misinformation about the disease. They were battles that never seemed to end. As late as 1961, Stein complained that a dermatologist told colleagues at a meeting of the Chicago Dermatological Society about the "excellent description of leprosy" in the Bible, a description the doctor said he could not "improve upon."[12]

By the time Brand met him in person, Stein was no longer the robust figure he had once been. The Hansen's bacilli had wreaked havoc on his body over the previous decades. He was not only blind, but his face, hands, and feet were covered in ulcers and scars, just the kind of damage that Brand was working so hard to eliminate. Stein was starting to show resistance to the sulfone drugs, so doctors had recently put him on an antibiotic called streptomycin. Unfortunately, one of the side effects was deafness. Stein, who had already lost his senses of sight and touch, was now losing his hearing as well. He found it increasingly difficult to hear the radio, recorded books, and conversations with friends, his last remaining links to the world in which he had once been so engaged. He told one visitor, "I did not know how fortunate I was when I was only blind."[13]

Brand still enjoyed chatting with Stein whenever he could. He admired the *Star* editor's intellect and passion, and the two would talk about the state of leprosy around the world. But such conversations became increasingly difficult. When Brand entered Stein's room, he would have to grab his hand and shake it vigorously before Stein realized that the doctor was there. Stein then put on his hearing aid and Brand would shout into it to communicate. Eventually, even that stopped working. Brand found it almost unbearable to watch as Stein's mind began to shut down. One day, he came in to find the ailing patient sitting in a chair, muttering to himself, "I don't know where I am. Is someone in the room with me? I don't know who you are, and my thoughts go round and round. I cannot think new thoughts."[14]

Stein could no longer use his hands, but his fingerprints were everywhere. The November–December 1967 issue of *The Star* was filled with stories that reflected his life's work. The paper reported that almost all of Carville's 125 registered voters had cast ballots in the November elections. Medal of Freedom holder and Filipina spy Joey Guerrero, who left Carville in 1957, had just become a U.S. citizen. Nearly one hundred golfers participated in the thirty-second semi-annual Carville invitational golf tournament. A nationally known quartet called the Diamonds was signed up to perform at that year's Christmas party. The paper also reprinted a letter chastising syndicated columnists Rowland Evans and Robert Novak for opening a recent column with the following sentence: "President Johnson's enthusiasm for a meeting with Soviet Premier Kosygin seems to be about the same as if he had been invited to a leper colony." The letter writer told the columnists that, on the contrary, Johnson—with whom Stein had once shared a stage in Texas—was no more likely to shun a leprosarium than he would any other hospital. The president had even issued a statement earlier that year bemoaning "the misplaced stigma attached to leprosy." Using words that could easily have been written by Stein, Johnson said, "Too many are unaware that often the disease can be cured, that deformity can be prevented and that rehabilitation can lead to self-sufficiency and society's welcome."[15]

As that issue of *The Star* was going to press, the longtime editor in chief was in the infirmary for blood transfusions. As sick as he was, Stein continued to work from his bed, dictating letters to contacts in Africa, Japan, and India. He was also busy making transition plans for *The Star*. He knew that his days were numbered and wanted to make sure that someone would carry on his life's work. Ironically, the progress Stein had fought so hard to achieve had made it more difficult to publish *The Star*. Newspaper staff turnover was higher than ever as patients responded positively to treatment and were quickly discharged. Stein suggested to hospital administrators that they set up a three-patient editorial board or a professional training program to ensure there would be someone available to take his place.[16]

On the morning of December 18, Stein was dictating letters to an assistant when he mentioned that he was not feeling well. The assistant suggested he take a break. "Very well," Stein responded. "Be here at ten tomorrow."[17] Stein died later that day, at age sixty-eight, almost four decades after Sidney Maurice Levyson first walked through the front gate with his monogrammed luggage.

News of Stein's death resonated far beyond the Carville community. His obituary was carried in newspapers across the country and noted in both *Newsweek* and *Time* magazines.

The Star received condolence letters from far and wide, including from Tallulah Bankhead. "Stanley was the bravest man I ever knew. I have lost a great friend," she wrote.[18]

Patients, staff, and guests gathered in the Protestant chapel for an ecumenical funeral service, before Stein's body was taken to San Antonio to be buried near where he was born. "The attitudes and the feelings of people both with the disease and without the disease are clearer and better today because of this man," said Merlin Brubaker, the current medical director. "The disease that for so long in history has confounded fact with fantasy does so less today because of Stanley Stein."

The official cause of death was kidney failure, with some signs of congestive heart failure. But Hansen's disease had taken its toll. Stein had volunteered for many experimental treatments over the years, but none was able to completely eliminate the effects of the *Mycobacterium leprae*. Still, the medical and social prospects for those entering the hospital were much better now, in part due to him. On the cover of the next issue of *The Star*, beneath its twenty-seven-year-old slogan, "Radiating the Light of Truth on Hansen's Disease," was a full-page picture of Stein. He's sitting at his desk, wearing a white shirt and dark tie, his eyes concealed by sunglasses resting on his thickened nose. His crippled hands are discreetly hidden, one beneath his chin and the other behind an arm. A nameplate on the desk says, "Mr. Stanley Stein, Editor." The caption below reads, "There is still much to be done. . . ."[19]

———

It was the late 1960s and the world was undergoing rapid change. The first African American had been appointed to the U.S. Supreme Court. A South African doctor had successfully transplanted a human heart. Three American astronauts had orbited the moon. Protests for gender and racial equality had erupted across the globe, sometimes accompanied by violence, but always propelled by a confidence that things could improve. Humanity was entering an exciting new era, one in which many believed they could shape their futures, if only they tried.

But in Laredo, Texas, a young man and his family were stuck in a distant past. Nineteen-year-old José Ramirez suffered from painful sores over large parts of his body and numbness in his fingers and forearms. He was so insensitive to pain that he would intentionally shock his twelve siblings by sticking needles into his arms without flinching. At the same time, other parts of his body were so hypersensitive he could barely tolerate the touch of his bedsheets. Ramirez was miserable, but no one knew why. His parents were beside themselves with worry and were running low on funds. They had used most of their limited savings seeking medical help for José, with little to show for it. One doctor told them their son had "grease balls" and he cut into the sores to drain them, hoping that would solve the problem, which it didn't. Another doctor said that José suffered from varicose veins and even operated on him, with no improvement. Another suggested his pain was imaginary.[20]

Frustrated, José's parents decided to seek help from the folk healers who were a traditional source of care in their Mexican American border community. If the professional doctors couldn't figure out what was wrong with their son, maybe the nonprofessionals could. These healers employed a combination of prayer, magic, and centuries of accumulated knowledge about the curative powers of plants. Some of the healers were effective, others were quacks, but the Ramirezes had nowhere else to go. As devout Catholics, they were used to relying on faith.

So in February 1967, José and his parents walked through a cold drizzle to the front door of a brick house in Nuevo Laredo, Mexico, a small town right over the border. Inside, they found a heavyset woman lying in bed, surrounded by several small children, velvet portraits of Jesus Christ on the walls. José sat on a wooden chair next to the bed, as the woman examined one of his hands. She told him his suffering was due to a long-ago breakup with a girl, who had probably put a curse on him as revenge. José was skeptical, but he watched his parents nod in agreement. The woman told them she needed to take José into the next room to pray, although he would have to do it in the nude. José, who didn't want to disappoint his parents, agreed. Surrounded by hundreds of lit candles, burning incense, and a picture of Our Lady of Guadalupe, José disrobed and the woman gently touched him from his head down to his feet. She said she was transferring the curse placed on him to herself. When she was done, José got dressed and rejoined his parents. His mother shed tears of joy, hopeful they had finally found the answer. His father sighed with approval, but José felt no better than before.

His was the plight of many Hansen's disease victims. It could take months, even years, to get a proper diagnosis. Doctors in America seldom encountered the disease and were easily confused. Symptoms varied greatly from patient to patient and were often similar to those of other ailments, such as syphilis, diabetes, allergies, and arthritis. Patients could be subjected to years of ineffective treatments before it was finally determined they had Hansen's disease. By then, it was more difficult to treat, and the patient was more likely to suffer permanent damage. That's what was happening to José Ramirez, whose young body was slowly being overtaken by the Hansen's bacilli, as doctor after doctor failed to catch the signs of leprosy.

José's parents continued their desperate search, seeking help from other folk healers, including a man who claimed to be an herbalist, or *yerbero*, although the Ramirezes were immediately suspicious. His "office" was in a rundown house on an unpaved road surrounded by vacant lots. The man asked for his payment up front, then took off his two-inch-wide belt, ordered José to remove his shirt, and started striking him on the back, with a promise that the "evil spirits would soon be beaten out" of the young man's body. José tried to bear the pain in silence as the man hit him again and again. But José's father, who was on the Laredo police force at the time, shouted, "Enough!" He pulled out his handgun and pressed it against the man's temple. "I will kill you if you strike him one more time."[21]

The Ramirezes decided it was time to give mainstream medicine another try. They took José to a doctor in San Antonio, who called himself a "world-renowned dermatologist." But he, too, failed to identify the disease. By December, José was having a hard time breathing and was extremely fatigued as he struggled through his classes at Laredo Junior College. A family friend finally convinced the Ramirezes to return to Mexico for help. This time, they went to see a folk healer in a small hut in an extremely poor neighborhood of Monterrey. It took only a few minutes for the elderly man to conclude that he could not cure José. "This disease is found in the Bible," he said, without mentioning the name. He told the family that José should be seen by a specialist who dealt with such diseases and suggested an anti-inflammatory drug called prednisone to ease his pain and discomfort.[22]

José and his parents left confused and discouraged, unaware that they had just received the most accurate diagnosis so far. A couple of months later, José lay in Mercy Hospital in Laredo, too weak to walk. Someone finally decided to send a sample of his skin tissue to the Public Health Service hospital in Carville for testing, and he soon got the devastating results. José was upset and confused; his parents were distraught. Leprosy was a disease they knew mostly from the Bible as a sign of an "unclean" soul, a symptom of sin. His parents did not blame José but themselves. They believed they had done something to offend God and were now being punished through the sufferings of their son. José's mother would tell him for decades that St. Peter would not let her into heaven because she had made him "unclean." Still, José was luckier than most. Unlike many people who are told they have leprosy, his family circled around in support. They hugged José and vowed to get him the best treatment they could. His girlfriend, Magdalena, stuck by his side, despite her mother's pleas that she end the relationship. The doctors at the hospital advised José to go to Carville, where, they said, he could be helped and possibly cured.

The first challenge was finding a way to get there. It was a 750-mile trip, sometimes along rough, narrow roads. José was in such pain he could not sit up, so the state health department's station wagon was out of the question, and no ambulances were available. His parents finally rented the only vehicle they could find—a hearse. At 4 a.m. a few days after his diagnosis, José was wheeled on a stretcher through the hospital, in what appeared to be a funeral procession. He was trailed by his sisters, his father, and his mother, who cried as she clutched her rosary beads. A priest followed, holding a Bible and praying as though he were about to administer the last rites. José saw hospital workers in face masks clinging to the walls as he rolled past. He was too sick to notice that he was put in a hearse and would not learn about his unusual mode of transportation for another ten years.

José's parents, one of his sisters, and his girlfriend got in a car to accompany the hearse on the nineteen-hour trip. José's sister, who worked in a hospital lab, administered morphine to ease his pain as they drove through countless small towns into the unknown. It was dark when they finally crossed the bridge over the Mississippi River into Baton Rouge and rolled past the towering Louisiana State Capitol and the LSU football stadium. They continued for twenty more miles, along dark, winding roads, before they finally reached Carville. The hearse brought José up to the back of the infirmary, where he was unloaded on a stretcher and rolled down a long hallway, like a body headed for the morgue. But Sister Victoria, the nurse who admitted him, kissed José on the forehead and assured him he would be okay. Times had changed and he was not asked to take an alias, although he would still have a number. He would be patient Number 2855. Technically, José was entering the hospital "voluntarily," but he would be unable to leave without a doctor's permission. He was told he might be home in as little as six months, but he would end up staying at Carville for the next ten years.

Chapter 19

Discrimination

IT WAS COMMON practice at Carville for older patients to take younger ones under their wing, like surrogate parents. Many children and young adults were on their own, having been abandoned by their families. José Ramirez's parents and siblings were exceptionally supportive of him, but they lived hundreds of miles away and could not afford to visit him often. So Darryl Broussard and his wife, Mary Ruth, informally adopted the young man and before long were calling him "son."

The Broussards had both come to Carville in 1939. Mary Ruth, twenty years old at the time, was picked up at her home in San Antonio, Texas, by a sheriff's deputy who told her he couldn't handcuff her because he was not allowed to touch her.[1] When she got to Carville, she was shocked to discover that her older sister was already there. Mary Ruth had been told by her parents that her sister was attending college in New Orleans—another family lie to cover up an embarrassing truth.[2] Darryl came from Lafayette, Louisiana, where he had grown up dreaming of playing football for LSU. Instead, he was taken to Carville and never returned home. Mary Ruth and Darryl eventually fell in love and were married. They did not have children of their own, so they were more than happy to keep an eye on Ramirez and gave his parents frequent updates on how their son was doing. They tried to make sure the young man stayed focused on his studies and his health, and didn't get into too much trouble now that he was on his own.

Indeed, there were many ways young men and women could get into trouble at Carville. There were plenty of rules to keep the patients confined, but those rules were frequently broken and by the 1960s almost everyone seemed to be in on the charade. The doctors and nurses knew that the place could explode if the patients didn't get to let off some steam now and then. One young woman said she loved to go out dancing and once was crawling through the hole in the fence (reopened after Dr. Gordon's departure) when her blouse snagged on a wire. As she struggled to get free, she saw one of Carville's physicians driving by. "I just waved," she recalled. She had little choice. The doctor waved back and drove on.[3]

Breaking the rules also made patients feel they had at least some control over their lives. They knew that many of the rules imposed on them were foolish, and existed more to ease public anxiety than anything else. Darryl, who ran the patients' post office, had his own form of protest. He was supposed to sterilize the outgoing mail, a practice that continued long after doctors recognized that it was unnecessary and perpetuated harmful myths about the disease. Dr. Johnwick groused at one point that the practice was "based on medieval rituals and custom that has its roots in the soil of ignorance" and should be stopped.[4] But he was overruled by the postmaster general, who worried about the impact on the nation's mail system if people learned that unsterilized letters from leprosy patients had been mixed in with their own. So Darryl routinely put sacks of mail in a small oven that produced noise and smoke but no sterilization. It was all for show, to make outsiders feel better, and the practice was finally ended in 1968.[5]

The younger patients defied the authorities in more adventurous ways. They often headed to the Red Rooster, a one-room bar with a tin roof about a mile down the river road, for a night of drinking, dancing, and dice games and, sometimes, a bar fight. One time, two brothers who were both patients got into an altercation at the Red Rooster and shot each other. They had to be taken to a nearby hospital before they were eventually returned to Carville.[6]

Another, more exclusive, club was located across the street from the leprosarium on the far side of the thirty-foot levee that protected the property from the volatile river. Several male patients had built their own private party house down by the water, out of sight of the guards. It was a small wooden hut, painted in rainbow colors, called the Ponderosa. The men kept rifles there to hunt squirrels and raccoons. They also grew and smoked marijuana, claiming it was for "medicinal" purposes. Most important, the Ponderosa was a place where male patients could share their most intimate stories, and even cry, without being judged. For those stuck in the institution across the street, the Ponderosa was a much-needed refuge, not unlike the shack that John Early and his fellow veterans had gathered in decades earlier.

Not too long after he arrived, when his worst symptoms had eased, José Ramirez was invited to join some of the other men for an evening at the Ponderosa. It was his first trip through the hole in the fence and after crossing the street and climbing the levee, he got his first view of the Mississippi River. He was stunned by its magnificence, with the opposite bank almost a mile away, and the muddy, powerful water rushing past. A bonfire was burning outside the hut, where several men sat drinking beer and smoking. Ramirez joined in, enjoying his first real chance to relax since coming to Carville. Suddenly, he spotted a police car rolling toward them along the top of the levee. He jumped up and started to look for a place to hide. But the other men just laughed and waved at the car. The sheriff's deputy was a friend checking to make sure they were all okay. Still, Ramirez was so unnerved that he decided to be more careful about future excursions.[7]

Mr. Pete was one of the other old-timers who helped Ramirez adjust to life at the hospital. He was among the patients who had been transferred to Carville from the Virgin Islands but never returned home. His job now was pushing wheelchair-bound patients around the complex. His hands were partially crippled, but reconstructive surgery had given him limited use of his thumbs and fingers, enough to grab the wheelchair handles and take new-comers where they needed to go. Mr. Pete's congenial personality also made him a good companion and informative guide. He loved Carville, especially because he knew how much better off he was there than if he'd stayed at the leprosy hospital in St. Croix.[8] Mr. Pete took his job very seriously, and wore a matching hat and suspenders as he rolled his charges down the long walkways from one appointment to the next. He was one of the first people Ramirez met at Carville. The young Texan's case had been left undiagnosed so long that he required intensive therapy when he first arrived. Mr. Pete took him to the clinic, where his feet and legs were soaked in warm water, covered in petroleum jelly, and wrapped in gauze to help his lesions heal and avoid infection.

Mr. Pete also gave him his first, and perhaps most useful, piece of advice. Ramirez had naïvely agreed to participate in a training session to help visiting professionals learn more about the disease. Mr. Pete warned him, as he wheeled him to the meeting room, not to say too much. "They don't care how we feel," he said. The wisdom of those words became instantly clear when Ramirez entered the meeting room and a doctor, without telling him what was about to happen, helped him to a standing position and, in front of twenty strangers, pulled the young man's pants and boxers down to his ankles to reveal his lesion-covered body. Ramirez was furious and embarrassed, but was too shocked to say anything. After it was over, as he waited in the hallway to be picked up by Mr. Pete, he vowed never to let himself be used that way again.[9]

It was a lesson that served Ramirez for many years. He realized that as much as doctors and nurses at Carville cared for the patients, they could also be patronizing and insensitive at times. The hospital provided some of the best medical treatment for Hansen's disease patients in the world, but the staff did not always see them as equals. It was partly a function of class. Many patients, like Ramirez, came from poor families, and increasing numbers of them were immigrants from Mexico and Asia. They had little in common with the highly trained specialists who now worked at Carville. It was also a time when those in authority still expected the people they served to be deferential.

In many ways, Ramirez was extremely fortunate. His girlfriend, Magdalena, stuck by his side and came to visit whenever she could. They made a handsome couple, she with a round, pretty face, and he with dark, curly hair, mustache, and goatee. During one of her visits, Ramirez, whose health was slowly improving, was given permission to take her to dinner at a restaurant in nearby Baton Rouge. As they were being seated, he spotted one of the hospital's top officials at a nearby table with his wife and some friends, and he decided to go over to greet them. But when the official saw his patient approaching, he quickly got up, intercepted him, and, as Ramirez recalled, "firmly grabbed my coat and sternly demanded to know what I was doing there, as if he owned the restaurant and I was not welcome." The young man returned to his table humiliated. Magdalena was furious. She pulled her boyfriend onto the dance floor and glared at the Carville official as she danced past him in the arms of the man she would eventually marry.[10] Long after Dr. Johnwick had declared that everyone at Carville was on the same team, patients were still treated like second-class citizens.

But this was the late sixties and revolution was in the air, even at Carville. José Ramirez was increasingly driven by the same fervor that motivated so many civil rights activists and protesters around the country. Authority was meant to be challenged and rules meant to be broken.

In the hot Louisiana summer, a swimming pool was a precious commodity. But at Carville only the staff had one, which the patients were strictly forbidden to use. It was another reminder that they were considered "unclean"—not unlike the many black children in the country at the time who were not welcome at so many community pools. After downing a couple of beers on one especially hot summer night, Ramirez and two of his friends decided it was time to defy the rules. They rode their bikes—the transportation of choice at Carville—to the staff side of the complex, their first violation. They then climbed over the chain-link fence that surrounded the pool, took off their clothes, and slipped into the forbidden water, luxuriating in its coolness on their embattled skin. They stayed for about an hour, two of them swimming beneath the moonlit sky, while the third young man clung desperately to the side of the pool; it turned out he did not know how to swim.[11] The three patients left undetected and satisfied that they had taken one small step toward breaking down the barriers that separated them from the rest of the world.

The patients were constantly reminded that those barriers still existed. On July 20, 1969, a group had gathered in the recreation center to watch, along with millions of people around the world, the first person walk on the moon. They were as excited as anyone to witness that "giant leap for mankind," until CBS news anchor

Walter Cronkite noted that officials were concerned the astronauts might pick up a disease on the moon that would require them to be quarantined. When Cronkite speculated that "leprosy might be one of those diseases," the Carville television was quietly turned off and the dispirited patients returned to their rooms. It was as if nothing had changed in the thirty years since patients felt compelled to turn off their radios when the World Series announcer described the umpire as the "leper" of the game. Humanity was about to achieve its greatest technological feat, but people with Hansen's disease were still seen as a threat.[12]

Ramirez soon learned that the world outside Carville and his small Texas community, where his illness drew sympathy from family and friends, could be extremely unkind to those with Hansen's disease. He enjoyed more freedom than earlier residents, because Carville's doctors were increasingly interested in integrating the patients into the community whenever they could. This meant that he was also far more exposed to the intolerance and ignorance of others. Ramirez was one of the first Carville patients allowed to enroll in nearby Louisiana State University. It took some maneuvering by the hospital's medical director to get LSU to accept a student who still tested positive for the disease, but to the university's credit, it finally agreed and Ramirez enrolled in the spring semester of 1969.

Ramirez was excited to continue his schooling, because he wanted to become a social worker. He bought a used Plymouth station wagon for $150 so he could commute to classes. But when he showed up for registration, Ramirez suddenly found himself in an alien world, alone in a "sea of white faces." When he approached a table promoting one of the fraternities, the student manning the desk pointed him toward a group of Indian students and said, "Your kind is over there."[13]

School became even more uncomfortable for him when word got out that a student at LSU had leprosy. *The Star* had published an article about Ramirez—without identifying him by name—and a national newspaper reprinted a condensed version under the headline "Leper Attends School at LSU." Someone at the university saw the article and posted a copy on a campus wall with a warning written beneath: "Beware, this guy may be in your class—shoot him."[14]

No one knew that Ramirez was the patient described in the article, but he was compelled to reveal his identity one day in a class entitled Social Problems. His professor was using leprosy patients as an example of one such problem, saying that "lepers" were a curse on society because they generated such high medical costs. He then joked that they also imposed a "cost to the clergy for making them bells for their necks." The other students laughed, but Ramirez was furious. He blurted out that people with Hansen's disease were neither "lepers" nor "social problems." When the startled professor asked what made him such an expert, Ramirez said it was because he was a "leper"—the only time he had ever used the word that he and the other patients despised. Ramirez saw some of the nearby students start to pull their desks away from him. But the professor not only apologized, he asked Ramirez to tell the class more about the disease and his experiences at Carville. The professor eventually visited the hospital and became a supporter, using the patients as an example in future classes of those in society who faced discrimination.[15]

Ramirez was again reminded of his outcast status when he later gave a group of LSU students a tour of the hospital. This time the discrimination came from inside the complex. The students stopped to have lunch in the staff dining room and Ramirez began to excuse himself because patients were not allowed to eat there. When one of the students asked why he was not joining them, Ramirez decided it was time to break another rule. The Carville cafeteria workers were not happy about it. One of them pulled Ramirez aside and told him he needed to go to the patient dining hall. The workers were worried they might get fired if they served him. They were African Americans and understandably did not want to lose what were considered very good jobs for blacks living in the South at the time. Ramirez decided to stay anyway, and the kitchen workers served him reluctantly, "their hard stares . . . telling me that their jobs might be in jeopardy," he later wrote.[16]

One irony was that Ramirez himself was the target of racial discrimination when he started to take a new medication. Some patients showed a resistance to dapsone, the main sulfone drug being used at the time. So the doctors were experimenting with a combination of drugs, hoping that if one medicine did not kill the germ in a particular patient, the others would. The latest addition to the mix was clofazimine, which had an unfortunate side effect. It turned skin dark—black and blue, almost purple, as though the patient had been beaten in a brawl. After he started taking the drug, Ramirez said that he was refused service at local stores and was stopped more frequently by the police. He wasn't called just a "leper" but also "boy" and "nigger."

There was one barrier that irked Ramirez more than any other. The Sacred Heart Catholic Chapel had served the spiritual needs of patients, staff, and visitors at Carville for more than thirty-five years. The red-brick church, behind the mansion, was shaped like a cross and had brilliant stained-glass windows. Several of the windows depicted the miracles of Christ, with the intentional omission of the one in which he cured the "lepers." One window displayed the words of Christ, including his promise to "console them in all their afflictions." The chapel was supposed to be a place where all could worship God together.

Yet it had three separate entrances. Visitors and staff were allowed to use two of them—the main door, in the center, and another one to the right of the altar. The patients had to use a separate entrance on the left. They also had to sit in their own section, apart from the rest of the congregation. When it was time for communion, staff and visitors went to one side of the altar, and the patients went to the other. The priest also used separate chalices for distributing the wafers that represented the body of Christ. There were even separate confessionals. One local man recalled that as a child he regularly attended Mass at the chapel with his mother, who worked in Carville's cafeteria. When they got home each Sunday, she would scrub him down with rubbing alcohol.[17] The message could not have been clearer. Patients were unclean and a danger to those around them.

Ramirez thought that if there was one place where people should be treated as equals it was in church. So one Sunday in early 1970, he decided to take a stand. Instead of using the side entrance, Ramirez walked up the front steps of the chapel and through the main door. He went down the center aisle, turned right, and sat in a front-row pew next to one of the hospital's surgeons. The rest of the congregation stared in shock. Up at the altar, the priest's face reddened but he proceeded to conduct the service as if nothing had changed. When it was time for communion, Ramirez stood up and followed a row of sisters up to the altar and knelt down beside them. On his other side was the surgeon, who repeatedly cleared his throat and nudged Ramirez with his elbow as the priest advanced along the rail to distribute the wafers. When he finally reached Ramirez, the priest hesitated, then, "in a reluctant manner, slowly moved his hand towards me with the host between his right thumb and index finger," Ramirez recalled. "I said, 'Amen,' and one of the decades-long practices at Carville came to an end."[18]

When Mass was over, a triumphant Ramirez crossed the church and went out the patients' doorway, expecting to be applauded by his fellow residents. Instead, he was met with silence. No one even made eye contact. As much as they might have agreed with Ramirez in principle, Carville patients were still reluctant to rock the boat. Many of them relied on Carville as their home and did not want to risk losing it. As Stanley Stein had learned decades earlier when he challenged the "leper" Mass, the Church was inviolable in this predominately Catholic community. Defying the authorities in such a way was seen as extremely foolish. The Broussards told Ramirez as much when he joined them for lunch at their Cottage Grove house several weeks later, and Darryl said grace. "Lord, thank you for giving us life and happiness on this planet and forgive us when we act stupidly in your house," he prayed. Ramirez learned his lesson.

————

Hanging over Carville like the oppressive heat of a Louisiana summer was the increasing possibility that the leprosarium might close. More than three hundred patients still lived there, but the federal deficit was growing and agencies were under pressure to cut costs. In 1970, the Public Health Service proposed shutting eight of its eleven hospitals around the country, arguing that the same medical care could be provided more economically at regular hospitals. Carville was not on the list, but it was only a matter of time.[19] As the drug therapy gradually became more effective, treatment of Hansen's disease patients at outpatient clinics was becoming increasingly feasible. Such clinics had already opened in California and New York and more of them were planned.[20] These were welcome developments for many of those who lived at the leprosarium, but not for all. Many longtime patients were understandably worried about their futures. Where would they go?

Even Paul Brand, the doctor who did such groundbreaking work on the effects of pain loss, was nervous about the impact of federal belt-tightening. It was becoming harder for him and other researchers at the hospital to justify spending money to help so few Americans. While twenty million people around the world suffered from Hansen's disease in the 1970s, only a few thousand lived in the United States. Fortunately, Brand discovered another benefit of his work that would end up helping millions of other Americans and secure his budget, at least for a while. He realized that people with diabetes, like those with Hansen's disease, were insensitive to pain because of damaged nerves. Brand believed that these patients, too, inadvertently damaged their feet by failing to take care of injuries that they did not know they had. His theory was initially dismissed by diabetes experts, until one of the top physicians in the field decided to survey his patients to see if Brand might be on to something. It turned out that, unbeknownst to that doctor, many of them had had their toes and feet amputated because of untreated cuts and infections. The discovery led doctors around the country, and eventually the world, to start checking diabetes patients' feet at every visit for signs of ulcers. Brand also opened Carville's foot clinic to people in the area who had diabetes and before long he was treating more of them than people with Hansen's disease.[21]

There was other groundbreaking research at Carville that helped to keep the budget cutters at bay. In 1968, Dr. Harry Burchfield, of the Gulf South Research Institute in New Iberia, Louisiana, answered an ad looking for someone to conduct studies on the use of dapsone, which was encountering more and more resistance among patients. Charles Shepard, the Public Health Service microbiologist who had succeeded in growing *Mycobacterium leprae* in the footpads of mice, came to discuss the project. He mentioned as an aside how difficult it was to duplicate the bacilli in the lab and that scientists had yet to find an animal that had the disease. Burchfield's wife, biochemist Eleanor Storrs, happened to be sitting in on the meeting. Her area of research involved armadillos, the curious-looking creatures common in the South. Storrs wondered aloud if armadillos might be suitable hosts for Hansen's disease. Their body temperatures were cool—something that was conducive to growing the bacilli—and they had life spans of twelve to fifteen years, which would give the slow-growing germ plenty of time to duplicate. Armadillos also gave birth to quadruplets, which would allow researchers to study the link between heredity and susceptibility to the disease.

As Storrs recalled, the other doctors initially laughed at her suggestion. They thought it was farfetched, and in truth, so did she. Repeated attempts to infect dogs, monkeys, guinea pigs, turtles, frogs, alligators, cats, parrots, and other animals had failed. But Storrs thought it was worth a try and pressed ahead. She eventually received a grant to work with doctors at Carville to test her theory.[22] Over the next year and a half, they inoculated forty-four armadillos, one of which, in the summer of 1971, died of the disease.

Researchers at Carville and elsewhere were ecstatic. It was the first time in history that leprosy had been detected in an animal other than humans. The discovery greatly expanded the opportunities scientists would have to study the disease and to search for better ways to treat, detect, and prevent it.[23] Before long, workers at Carville were rounding up wild armadillos and bringing them to the former dairy barn behind the cemetery to be used for research. The animals were kept in wooden pens with piles of cut-up paper from old issues of *The Star* to use for burrowing.[24] Patients, including José Ramirez, also began catching the animals so they could earn extra money selling them to researchers for five dollars apiece.

Doctors used the armadillos not only to learn more about the disease but to produce millions of bacilli to be sent to researchers around the world. The goal was to find out exactly how leprosy was spread—which was still a mystery—and whether a vaccine could be developed. In 1975, Carville received a $95,288 government grant to support its armadillo colony. Scientists would eventually conclude that not only could they infect armadillos with the disease but that armadillos could also give it to humans. A certain strain of Hansen's disease bacilli was found in both humans and armadillos in areas where the animals were a popular source of meat, such as Brazil. It was unclear how the armadillos got the disease—some scientists believed the animals picked up the germ digging in the dirt, but no one was sure. One thing was clear. Eleanor Storrs had given Carville's supporters another argument against closing the doors of a place that had caused great sorrow over the years but also provided extraordinary comfort and hope.[25]

On August 25, 1977, a small, painfully shy Vietnamese girl was brought to the front gates of Carville by a young Vietnamese man. They had driven down from Dallas, where a few days earlier the girl had been diagnosed with Hansen's disease. Her face was swollen—almost twice its normal size—and her skin was mottled with lesions. The girl, Mien Pham, was eleven years old, although her doctor had told a local newspaper she was nine.[26] Mien probably looked younger than she was because she was almost certainly malnourished.

Mien was among tens of thousands of South Vietnamese citizens who had fled Saigon in the spring of 1975 as North Vietnamese troops descended upon the city. She worked as a nanny and servant for a wealthy family, but in truth she was more like a slave. Her parents were extremely poor and had given her to the family when she was only six years old so she could have a better life, or so they hoped. Her job was to care for the family's two young sons—who were only slightly younger than she was—in exchange for food and a place to live. Instead, she was often beaten and starved.

Mien held the boys' hands tightly as they scrambled with the mass of refugees to board an American ship waiting in Saigon's harbor to take them away. Mien was terrified as they leaped from a bouncing barge to a platform on the ship. She knew that if they slipped between the two, they would die. But they made it and were quickly pulled up a rope ladder to the deck above.[27]

In the chaos of flight, the three children were separated from the boys' mother and their uncle, the young man who would eventually bring Mien to Carville. The American ship took the children to Guam, where they lived for months until they were reunited with the rest of the family. From there, they were moved to the Fort Chaffee army base in Arkansas and finally resettled in an apartment outside Dallas. For Mien, little changed at first. She was still beaten by the mother and forbidden to eat with the rest of the family. "I was always so hungry," she said many years later. She sometimes tried to sneak food out of the refrigerator when no one was watching, but if she was caught, she was beaten. Other times, desperate, she would search behind the couch cushions for spare change to buy food. Once, the boys' mother mistakenly gave her a ten-dollar bill to buy groceries, thinking she was giving her a five. Mien used some of the change to buy a large candy bar that she could eat quickly. She saved the rest of the money to buy more food later.

One thing about her new life was better. In America, Mien was required to go to school, something she loved to do. She got plenty of food there and nobody hit her. But the school nurse noticed one day that Mien had an odd rash and bumps on her face and insisted that the family take her to a doctor. After testing her skin, the doctor informed the family that Mien had leprosy and recommended that she be taken to a special hospital in Louisiana.

At first, it was scary. She was far from home, alone, and confused. But Mien soon realized that Carville was the best place she had ever lived. "It was like heaven." There was plenty to eat and people were kind. "I looked just like everybody else and nobody was scared of me." Mien liked Carville so much that she was distraught when she was sent back to Dallas after a month of treatment, something that was done because doctors at the time believed it was best for young patients to be cared for at home whenever possible. But Mien only got sicker there. She was once again starved, and she was forced to stay inside. The family did not want anyone to know she was back home. Mien was given her own set of dishes and utensils and was not allowed on the furniture. She could sit on the floor only if she covered it with newspaper.

When Mien returned to Carville for more treatment, she told the doctors she did not want to go home. Eventually, she was allowed to stay, but she still struggled with the disease. Like José Ramirez, she was put on clofazimine, which made her skin appear black and blue. Her face and arms were also mottled with bumps. Once, around 1984, when she went to visit a friend in San Francisco, a man in an elevator looked at her face and remarked, "It's not Halloween yet." Mien burst into tears.

Mien lived at Carville until she was discharged at the age of twenty-two. She married a Carville employee and they built a home in nearby Gonzales on an expanse of land that they filled with fruit trees and flower gardens. Sometimes they invited their Carville friends, including the Daughters of Charity, to join them for cookouts. Mien and her husband were married for ten years, until he died in a car crash on his way to work. After his death, she decided to go to Texas to see the Vietnamese family that had treated her so cruelly. She wanted to let them know that she had turned out okay. She had already sent them a basket of fruit from her yard as a gift. But the family refused to open the door.

Mien believed that Carville had saved her life, not only by healing her wounds but by rescuing her from a troubled life. To her it was the opposite of prison; it was freedom. By the 1980s, that's what the hospital had become for many of the patients, a haven from what could still be a cruel life for those with Hansen's disease. They were not about to give that up.

Chapter 20

Shutting Down

THE PRESSURE TO close Carville was building. The new Reagan administration swept into office in 1981 promising to shrink the government, and the leprosy hospital in Louisiana seemed like a good target. The government was spending $18 million a year to employ 450 full- and part-time staffers to care for about two hundred patients.[1] There were also ninety-eight buildings and sprawling grounds to maintain, which included keeping all those massive live oak trees pruned and alive.[2] It was an expensive place to run.

There were also medical reasons to close up shop. It's impossible to pinpoint the exact moment when Hansen's disease was "cured," but 1981 was the year when the world finally agreed on the most effective treatment. Dr. Faget's discovery at Carville in the 1940s that patients responded positively to promin was the first step, but it took decades of testing different combinations and doses of antibiotics to settle on one that seemed to work for the most patients. The best combination, it turned out, was dapsone, clofazimine, and another antibiotic called rifampin. This three-drug treatment was so effective at arresting cases and preventing reactivation that the World Health Organization recommended it as the preferred treatment worldwide. Most patients stopped being contagious after a few days of taking the drugs and their bodies could be completely free of *Mycobacterium leprae* within a year. The U.S. government was also in the process of setting up more outpatient clinics where those diagnosed with leprosy could be treated closer to home and hopefully avoid the permanent disabilities that often resulted from delayed care. There seemed to be fewer and fewer reasons to operate a massive, and expensive, facility in Louisiana.

The question was what to do with the patients who lived there. In September 1982, members of Congress came to Carville to hold a hearing on how a cost-saving plan to contract out medical services to private health-care providers would affect what was now called the National Hansen's Disease Center. In the middle of the dais sat California Democrat Henry Waxman, the short, balding chairman of the House Energy and Commerce Committee's Subcommittee on Health and the Environment. Waxman exerted oversize influence over national health policy. On either side of him were two of Carville's staunchest congressional supporters, Louisiana's Democratic congressman Gillis Long and congresswoman Lindy Boggs.[3] The witness list was stacked against the Republican administration's plan, although one official did testify that contracting out medical operations government-wide would save taxpayers a billion dollars a year.

Testimony against the plan was passionate and almost unanimous. Representatives of *The Star*, the Patients' Federation, the American Legion, the hospital staff, and local communities all saw the proposal as the first step toward shutting the hospital down. Witness after witness argued that Carville was a unique place that outsiders would not be able to understand, and Congressman

Long agreed. "The compassion that employees have here can't be purchased from a contractor," he said, adding that patients' health would suffer if the proposed change went into effect. Long and Boggs noted that the hospital provided much-needed jobs for local residents and even patients, and that important medical research would be lost. Witnesses also spoke emotionally about the obstacles patients would face if they were forced to leave. "You can imagine how tough it must be for victims of this disease and their families when many of them are forced to live in . . . constant fear that their secret will be discovered," the former head of the Patients' Federation told the lawmakers. The testimony seemed to work. Carville was spared from having its services contracted out, but it was clear to all that the leprosarium's days were numbered.[4]

One problem for those trying to preserve Carville was that leprosy was barely on anyone's radar. So few people got the disease in the United States anymore that most Americans were unaware that it still existed. Even fewer knew that their government ran a leprosarium and that patients, up until the 1960s, had been confined there against their will.

At the time of Waxman's hearing, people were much more alarmed about another mysterious illness, which was afflicting otherwise healthy homosexuals. Five young men had died suddenly in Los Angeles the year before from a rare lung infection. Dozens more had been diagnosed with a form of cancer called Kaposi's sarcoma. Most of the victims lived in California and New York, but by the end of 1981 about 130 individuals had died and gay men around the country were frantic. It appeared that all the victims had a severe immune deficiency and that whatever caused it was sexually transmitted. By 1982, there were warnings that tens of thousands of people might be affected by the viral disease, which was finally given a name, acquired immune deficiency syndrome, or AIDS.[5]

Doctors were perplexed and the public was understandably frightened. Some responded with suggestions similar to those made a century earlier when people were worried about other infectious diseases, including leprosy. Even some health professionals believed that AIDS victims should be isolated on islands or elsewhere to prevent the virus from spreading. These suggestions were eventually dismissed as unworkable and a violation of patient rights, but they were seriously contemplated. A Boston neurosurgeon, Dr. Vernon Mark, caused a stir in 1985 when he proposed that AIDS patients who behaved irresponsibly—in other words, continued to have sex—be quarantined on Penikese Island in Buzzards Bay, the same place where Massachusetts's leprosy patients had been isolated sixty years earlier, before they were shipped off to Carville. Mark insisted that he did "not want to create a new class of lepers" but said that current policies were failing. He also called for mandatory blood tests for those, particularly homosexuals, who were especially vulnerable to AIDS. Mark made his comments at a conference of political conservatives, who suggested that pornography was a major reason the disease was spreading.[6]

Because AIDS affected primarily gay men, the public's initial reaction was overwhelmingly homophobic. As with leprosy, this new illness was seen as a reflection of the victim's moral deficiency. The men who got AIDS deserved it because they engaged in "abnormal" sexual behavior, went the thinking of some. When intravenous drug users began to get the disease, there was a similar response. Those who did not engage in homosexuality or use drugs believed they were immune. One doctor, interning at a Bronx hospital in 1985, was alarmed to see another intern treating AIDS patients without wearing protective gloves. The intern confidently told him, "Don't worry, if you lead a clean life, you're not going to catch this disease."[7] As with leprosy, family members and friends abandoned victims of the disease because they feared both the contagion and humiliation.[8] Those infected with AIDS began to fear public exposure almost as much as the disease itself.

Attitudes began to change in 1984 when the disease hit a victim who was neither gay nor a drug user. Thirteen-year-old Ryan White, a hemophiliac, was infected when he received a transfusion of contaminated blood. The Indiana boy's case quickly became the symbol of public confusion over how to respond to this new epidemic. White insisted on returning to his middle school after he was diagnosed with AIDS, but more than 150 parents and teachers demanded that he be barred from classes. They feared he would infect the other children, even though doctors insisted the disease was not spread through casual contact. White's family sued the board of education and their son was finally allowed to attend classes, as long as he used disposable utensils and a separate restroom. Several families withdrew their children from the school and set up an alternative one, rather than risk exposure to the disease. White and his family were shunned and threatened. White's mother said passersby sometimes yelled at her son on the street, "We know you're queer." The family finally moved to another town after a bullet was shot through their living-room window.[9] It was as though the lessons of leprosy had never been learned.

Indeed, public intolerance of those with Hansen's disease had never gone away. In the spring of 1987, employees and patients at a health clinic in San Jose, California, threatened to quit and boycott if the facility agreed to treat people with leprosy. The clinic had been awarded a contract by the Public Health Service to serve as one of the outpatient facilities that were gradually replacing Carville. "I'd rather have them treat AIDS patients here than leprosy," one of the patients complained to a reporter. The clinic's switchboard operator, a mother of two boys, threatened to quit. "I don't want to be giving it to my children," she said. "Sure, they deserve to be treated," said another employee. "I just don't want them around my kids."

Roy Jimenez, a clinic official, was frustrated by the resistance. "There are more serious problems. AIDS, my goodness. Drug abuse. High-risk pregnancies. Battered wives. Negligence. Hansen's disease is just so benign," he told a reporter. "It pales in comparison to the big problems we have. But it's leprosy, and in people's minds, it creates a lot of fear." The proposal was eventually dropped and the clinic's operators found somewhere else in the San Francisco Bay area where those with Hansen's disease could go for care.[10]

On March 11, 1999, several dozen Carville patients and their supporters gathered by the front gate through which so many frightened and abandoned people had entered over the past century. They were getting ready to protest the latest effort to make them leave. It was quite a sight, with some patients sitting on wheelchairs, golf carts, and bicycles, and others standing with the help of crutches and canes. Some carried hand-painted signs; others had posters attached to their vehicles. "Carville is our home, leave us alone," read one sign. "You are stealing our home," "Why have you lied to us?" and "Heck no, we won't go," read others. Reporters and TV camera crews were there to record the event.[11]

At issue was the government's latest plan to shut down the hospital and return the property to the state of Louisiana. As far as federal health authorities were concerned, Carville had outlived its usefulness. Patients still went there temporarily for treatment, but no new long-term residents had been admitted for almost fifteen years and the hospital's research department had been moved to LSU. Several cost-sharing measures had been tried over the years to keep the center open and to appease patients who wanted to stay. But nothing seemed to work.

The most ambitious effort had been a flop. The government decided in 1991 to lease half of the facility to the U.S. Bureau of Prisons (BOP) to house minimum-security prisoners in need of long-term medical care.[12] The unusual arrangement—with about two hundred prisoners and an almost equal number of Hansen's disease patients sharing the same facilities—ended after three years.[13] It wasn't a good fit. Although the two groups rarely mixed, the Hansen's disease patients were happy to see the prisoners go. Their presence only reminded the patients that they were still seen as society's castoffs. Carville's Mardi Gras parade that year included a float with a patient posing as a corpse in a casket, with "RIP BOP 1991–1993" written on a fake tombstone. The float won the first-place prize.

In 1998, the federal government came up with another plan. It offered patients an annual $33,000 stipend for the rest of their lives if they would move out for good. Forty-five patients accepted the deal. Among them was Rachel Pendleton, who had lived at Carville for almost fifty years. She said the government had robbed her of the best years of her life. "I really want to get out of here and forget this place ever existed."[14]

But more than eighty other patients did not want to leave. Most of them were in their sixties, seventies, and eighties. None of them had Hansen's disease anymore—they had been cured years ago with the drug therapy—but they were frail or disabled and had become dependent on the hospital for care. The government promised that they could stay at Carville as long as they were ambulatory and could take care of themselves. If they were bedridden or required extensive care, they would be moved to a nursing facility in Baton Rouge. It sounded like a good deal, but after years of fighting the authorities, the patients were skeptical. They wanted a written guarantee that they could stay if that was what they chose to do. They signed a petition to President Bill Clinton asking for that assurance. "Honor our choice to live out our lives in this, the only home we have ever known." The patients noted that in coming to Carville they had been separated from their families once already and "forced to create a new family. . . . If we are moved as planned, we will be uprooted and once again separated from our families. . . . To do this to us a second time is not only cruel, but unjust."[15]

The protesters planned to parade from the front gate along what was now called Stanley Stein Drive, the main road that cut through the center of the property. They would pass the cream-colored infirmary and network of dorms on their right. On their left would be the modest houses where the remaining staff lived. As they approached Lake Johansen, they would turn right toward Cottage Grove, and stop at the cemetery, where hundreds of their fellow patients lay buried beneath rows of identical government-issued tombstones. It was sometimes called the "longest mile in the world," the journey from Carville's entrance to inevitable death. The cemetery seemed a fitting spot to make the point that Carville was where they should be allowed to live out their lives.

There were some familiar faces in the crowd as the marchers set off to the strains of "Don't Fence Me In," blaring from a boom box. Mr. Pete, who had been institutionalized since the age of six, led the parade on his bicycle. "We want to stay here until we die," he told a reporter. Eighty-one-year-old Mary Ruth Daigle, who had been a Carville resident since 1939, felt the same. "The government brought me here," she said. "I became a ward of the government, and I think they should take care of me till I die."[16]

Johnny Harmon was also there. He was now a frail eighty-seven-year-old who pedaled along on his large three-wheeled bike with a horn attached so he could alert pedestrians he was coming.

The octogenarian was slightly bent over but still had a thick head of white hair and a warm smile. Johnny and his wife, Anne, had returned to Carville in 1993 so they could be cared for in their old age, something longtime residents were allowed to do. It was an attractive deal for those who had lost so much of their lives. Harmon was not about to give it up now. "They'll have to take me out in a box," he said. Sadly, he would soon be alone; his wife died within days of the protest.[17]

José Ramirez, who had been discharged in 1976 and went on to become a social worker, was also there. He had become an international advocate for Hansen's disease patients and helped to organize the protest. Ramirez was joined on the march by ninety-year-old Betty Martin, who had returned to Carville with her husband Harry nine years earlier after more than four decades living on their own. The Martins never overcame the stigma of leprosy and the burden of keeping their past a secret. As their health deteriorated, mostly from old age, they decided to return to the one place where they felt secure and among friends.

Betty was now alone. Harry had died in 1996.[18] Betty was confined to a wheelchair but looked as elegant as ever, her gray hair neatly styled, nails manicured, and wearing makeup fit for a Louisiana debutante, as she was wheeled to the cemetery. She wore a wide-brimmed hat that protected her face from the sun, which suddenly emerged from the clouds just as the patients reached their destination. "This day is a beautiful day for victory," Betty remarked as she and Ramirez dug a hole next to one of the graves. In it they placed pieces of paper bearing the names of all the barriers they had faced in life but hoped could now be buried forever—"prejudices," "stigma," "labeling," "the 'l' word," "unfounded fear," and "emotional pain."[19]

Shortly after the protest, the patients received the written assurance they sought. The head of the Health Resources and Services Administration, which had taken over operation of the hospital from the Public Health Service, said patients would be allowed to stay at Carville as long as they were able to care for themselves. Otherwise, they would be moved to the nursing home in Baton Rouge, where they could remain for the rest of their lives. Almost sixty patients ultimately decided to stay at Carville and were there on April 8, 1999, when the property was finally returned to the state of Louisiana. The state planned to use the site as a National Guard base and a training facility for at-risk youth. Most of the old Carville buildings would be preserved as part of a National Historic Site. By 2001, the number of residents had dropped to thirty-eight, as patients either died or moved to Baton Rouge.[20] Betty Martin and Johnny Harmon both died at the nursing facility the following year. The Daughters of Charity finally closed their mission at Carville in 2005, their nursing services no longer required.

One of the few remaining patients was Perry Enriquez, who had returned from California in 1984 after his wife, Maria, died. He no longer suffered from Hansen's disease but was getting older and knew he would be cared for there until he died. At age seventy-five, Perry married another patient and they lived together at Carville for a quarter century more, enjoying their music and friends. Unlike in his first marriage, Perry and his second wife could come and go as they pleased. Perry was moved to the Baton Rouge nursing facility in 2010 shortly before his death at the age of 102.

Oscar Dempster, who had arrived when he was seven, died that same year at age ninety-one. His niece and her husband, who lived nearby, had invited Oscar years earlier to come live with them. But he preferred to stay where he was. For Perry and Oscar and many of the other longtime patients, Carville turned out to be a wonderful place to grow old. "He was happy there. What started out at the beginning as kind of a tragedy I guess, really turned out to be a good thing," said Perry's daughter, Dolores, one of the two little girls who used to take the ferry across the river to see their father. "It was the one thing the government got right. They fig-ured out they made a mistake and then they tried to correct it."[21]

All of the patients had moved out by 2015. Among the last to leave was Simeon Peterson, or Mr. Pete. He spent his final years at Carville working as a guide for the occasional visitors who stopped by to explore the small National Hansen's Disease Museum on the grounds and to learn about this unusual chapter in American his-tory. Mr. Pete could often be seen riding along the now-empty cor-ridors on his bike, wearing his signature suspenders and matching hat, probably more alone than he'd ever been in his life. He moved to the Baton Rouge nursing facility in 2014 and died there in 2017 from cancer. Mr. Pete had been institutionalized for eighty-three of his eighty-nine years for a disease that posed little threat to those around him. He outlived everyone in his family, and most of the people he had ever known.[22]

––––––––

The government's isolation of Hansen's disease victims left a trail of shattered families in its wake. The patients were rejected and isolated by society, but their children and spouses also suffered from exclusion and loss. The forced separation was worse when it was cloaked in secrecy—as it so often was—as though the loved one had committed a serious crime and the whole family had to live with the shame. Children, more than anyone else, seemed to bear the brunt of the pain.

Linda Williams was initially surprised and bitter when she was reunited with her mother in 1977. Surprised because she had forgotten how bigger-than-life her tiny mother was, with her three-inch heels and hair piled on top of her head like Marge Simpson, the cartoon character. The woman she met at the New Orleans air-port also had an unusually loud voice, calling out Linda's Japanese name as her Carville husband clicked away with his camera, trying to chronicle their reunification. "Wow, so this is my mother," Williams thought.[23]

Williams was bitter because her mother had left her with her American stepfather in Okinawa, Japan, when she was only seven years old. This was the first time she had seen her in fifteen years. For most of that time, Williams thought that her mother, Tetsuko Klockgether, had abandoned her. She did not know that Klockgether had Hansen's disease and was living at a hospital in Louisiana, or that she had gotten remarried. The young woman was also upset because, once she learned the truth, she did not understand why her mother had gone so far away when there were leprosaria in Japan. But Williams soon learned what many other relatives of Carville patients had come to recognize. Her mother was ashamed of her disease and did not want to embarrass her family. By going more than twelve thousand miles from home, she could keep her illness a secret, even if she had to leave her little girl behind.

Klockgether was thrilled when her daughter wrote and said she wanted to see her mother again. She told Williams that she thought about her every day they were apart. She also said that she had tried to kill herself a couple of times because she was so sad about leaving her daughter. Now that they were reunited, Williams invited her mother to come live with her and her husband in Michigan. But Klockgether, like so many of the other aging patients, did not want to leave Carville. She had a husband and friends there, and a job as an X-ray technician. Klockgether stayed at Carville until her death in 2014 at the age of eighty-six. She had found happiness there, although her daughter admitted that she herself had often felt insecure as a child, not knowing why her mother had left. "I'd rather just be in the shadow," Williams recalled.

Edmond Landry's granddaughter, Claire Manes, who wrote a book called *Out of the Shadow of Leprosy* about her family's experiences at Carville, felt similar anxieties as a child. She knew that her grandfather's illness was not to be discussed. Whenever she asked her mother or grandmother how her grandfather had died, the question was quickly brushed aside. She was simply told that he had died of kidney disease, which was true but hardly the whole story. "We just kind of knew not to talk about him," said Manes. She learned the truth when her mother pulled her aside after she and her younger brother had made some childish jokes about "lepers." Her mother said such jokes were hurtful and revealed that Manes's grandfather had had leprosy. They never mentioned it again, until decades later.[24]

In 1977—the same year that Linda Williams was reunited with her mother—Albert Landry, the last of the five Landry siblings, died at Carville. He had lived there for more than thirty-five years. His two sisters had already died, Amelie in 1940, and Marie, who arrived with Albert in 1941, in 1962. When relatives were clearing out Albert's room they came across a stash of letters, the ones that Edmond and Norbert had written a half century earlier. The discovery encouraged Manes to explore her grandfather's past in the hope of unraveling some of the mysteries that surrounded her childhood. She eventually asked her mother what it had been like to have her father taken away when she was only five years old. Her mother, Teenie, recalled how Edmond had kissed her goodbye and driven out of her life. Manes believed that the experience made her mother reserved and standoffish as an adult, but also more compassionate toward others who had troubled lives. But Teenie was also bitter about how her father was treated. "They told us it was contagious. It wasn't. They told us it was hereditary. It wasn't. They told us it was dangerous. It wasn't," she complained when, in her eighties, she finally began to talk about what had happened. Manes asked her mother how that made her feel. The elderly woman, who seldom swore, simply responded, "Like shit."

Manes said her brother believed that "the story of our family was that we did not tell stories." Her nephew, Christopher, did not think that the family was ashamed of Edmond or Norbert or their disease, but that having "had the lives of an entire generation just stripped away from them was too painful to discuss."[25] With the luxury of time and distance, Claire Manes wondered what life might have been like had there not been so much secrecy. "Perhaps all of us in the family would have been more generous with hugs, kisses, and physical affection had this unspoken taboo not hung over us." She imagined some of the things she might have done as a little girl if her grandfather had not been taken away. "It is pleasant to think that we would have walked along the family property, flown kites, and ridden horses in the pasture," she wrote. "He would have taught us to strip the cane in the fields and chew its long stalks. We would have picked pecans and peaches on the family property, caught crawfish that crawled out of their holes in the spring, or explored the attic at the home on Weeks Street. . . . We may have even walked with him to Estorge Drug Company where he worked and sipped fountain Cokes as we sat on chairs at the counter, our legs swinging."[26]

Harold Koll bore similar scars as an adult. More than six decades after his father, Morris, was taken to Carville, Harold called up his children to tell them the truth. He had held in the secret for too many years. Like Teenie and Linda Williams, Harold was quiet and reserved and often felt unsure of himself. He believed that the loss of his father was partly to blame. Harold became a meat salesman and never achieved the financial security his family had known before Morris was taken away. After visiting Carville for the first time in 1998, Harold told his children he thought he was a failure in life, although no one else agreed. He was the only one of his siblings to reveal his father's secret and to come to grips with this sad slice of America's past. He was also a gentle soul, who, having lost his father, held tightly to his children, grandchildren, and great-grandchildren.

For days after they came for visits, he would not allow his wife to clean their fingerprints off doors and walls.

John Early's family also suffered from his long and combative struggle with both the disease and its stigma. John and Lottie had three sons when she asked for a divorce. It's impossible to know what impact the separation had on the boys, but Early's great-granddaughter, Gina DeRose Bell, said two of the three were dead by the age of thirty. Emmanuel, the oldest, died in a car accident. Ralph Paul, the one born in the divided house along the Potomac River, took his own life. Bell said her mother described Lottie as "distrustful and aloof" and an erratic mother at best. Early's youngest son, Roy, told of coming home from school with his brother Emmanuel one day to discover that their mother and other brother had moved from their Oakland, California, home to Los Angeles, leaving them behind. The two boys found their way to San Francisco, where they lived with their stepfather—separated at the time from Lottie—until their mother returned the following year.

Bell never knew her great-grandfather John Early but was upset when she learned that he had been incarcerated and ostracized for much of his life. She believed that medical authorities, who knew better, should have done more to educate the public about Hansen's disease instead of forcing the patients to pay the price. Bell also saw parallels with the nation's response to AIDS and other diseases.[27] She recalled that a nurse was quarantined in New Jersey in 2014 after returning from Africa where she had worked with Ebola patients. The nurse was confined in a tent— just like Bell's great-grandfather was—even though she showed no signs of being sick and tested negative for Ebola.[28] Claire Manes said her elderly mother was similarly appalled by suggestions that AIDS patients should be secluded on islands. "She said, 'They can't do that!'" because she knew the pain it would cause.

Chapter 21

Lessons Not Learned

LEPROSY, OR HANSEN'S disease, still exists. About two hundred new cases are diagnosed in the United States each year; worldwide, there are about two hundred thousand new cases, mostly in India, Brazil, and Indonesia. Millions of people living today were diagnosed with Hansen's disease at some point in their lives. Most are now cured but almost three million people still struggle with disabilities, such as crippled hands and feet or blindness, the result of delayed diagnosis and care. Almost all victims at some point have faced the stigma of a disease that is still dreaded and misunderstood by much of the world.[1]

Surprisingly, doctors are still unsure how Hansen's disease is spread. In some ways, it remains as mysterious as ever, all these many decades after Gerhard Hansen first spotted those rod-shaped bacilli through his microscope lens in his lab in Bergen, Norway. Experts believe the germs are transmitted from one person to another in tiny droplets from the nose or mouth. Or, in some cases, from contact with an infected armadillo. What scientists know for certain is that leprosy is a mild threat to the world. An individual cannot get it through casual contact, and 95 percent of the human race is naturally immune. All that banishing and fumigating and locking in boxcars over the centuries was for naught.

Still, for those who do get Hansen's disease, the effects can be devastating without proper medical care. Researchers are still looking for a vaccine to prevent the disease from spreading and for a quick, simple diagnostic test, so it can be spotted and treated before permanent disabilities have a chance to set in.

There has been tremendous progress over the years fighting the disease. The World Health Organization, with the help of the Nippon Foundation and the pharmaceutical company Novartis, has been able to drastically reduce the number of cases worldwide, from about five million new ones in 1985 to a fraction of that today. They did this in part by offering, free of charge to anyone who needs it, the medication needed to cure the disease—the same multidrug therapy used at Carville of rifampin, clofazimine, and dapsone.

Despite all this, health officials have failed to achieve their ultimate goal of wiping Hansen's disease from the planet. Instead, the number of new cases has plateaued, with unsettling spikes here and there. Victims still face some of the same obstacles today that people have confronted for centuries. Patients are frequently misdiagnosed because medical professionals are unfamiliar with the disease. Many who become ill lack access to proper medical care. Others are too afraid to reveal that they're sick.

It comes down to this: All the medical knowledge in the world has failed to eliminate the biggest barriers to treating Hansen's disease—discrimination, superstition, and ignorance. The stigma of leprosy lives on. Even today about half of those who go to the National Hansen's Disease Program's outpatient clinic in Baton Rouge say they considered killing themselves after they were diagnosed. They were terrified that they would be ostracized and, despite repeated assurances from doctors, that they might never be cured. Some even believed that they deserved to be stricken, that it was God's way of punishing them for their sins. Their biggest fear was that others would discover they had the disease.

Patients have reason to be worried. Even in the twenty-first century, Hansen's disease victims can be reviled and discriminated against. Many are still isolated from family and friends. In India, leprosy was grounds for divorce until 2019. United Nations human rights experts complained the same year that children with Hansen's disease were denied schooling in Brazil.

Patients in the United States are not immune from the scorn. In the early 2000s, a couple returned home from the Baton Rouge clinic, where one of them had been treated, to discover that the rental house they lived in had been sold while they were away. The landlord was one of their parents. Another patient, upset by the reception she had received from relatives when she came home from the clinic, sought advice from a friend, who was a medical professional she thought she could trust. He was also on the local school board, and the woman was horrified later to discover that he was organizing a meeting of parents to warn them that one of the parents had leprosy. The only silver lining was that the woman's relatives were so angry at how she had been treated, they rallied around her in support.[2]

It seems that whenever the word *leprosy* is mentioned, people instinctively recoil. That was true in 1918, and it is still true over a century later. It's an exotic and alarming disease, if only in people's minds. When parents at an elementary school in Jurupa Valley, California, learned in 2016 that two students were suspected of having the disease, some of them pulled their children from classes. Others sent their children to school with masks covering their mouths. "It's just very, very scary," said one of the fathers.

Officials assured the parents that their children were safe, but several classrooms were disinfected just to be sure, not unlike what happened in Frank and Hale George's New Jersey school in 1925.[3]

Even medical professionals can be rattled by a disease they seldom encounter. Francisco Sanchez, a Carville patient in the late 1990s, recalled going to a hospital in California for a knee injury. When he gave his medical history, the doctor jumped away from him, explaining that leprosy was highly contagious. Sanchez suggested that the doctor might want to visit the Hansen's disease clinic two floors above and learn the truth.[4]

Current and former patients complain that stigma and prejudice follow them everywhere. José Ramirez notes that the words *leper* and *leprosy* are still commonly used to describe something abhorrent, as in 2014 when Pope Francis referred to pedophile priests as a "leprosy" on the Catholic Church. When I was writing this chapter, I decided to search for the most recent use of *leper* in the news and was horrified to discover it was on NPR, the radio network where I work. During an interview about failing start-up businesses, a guest commented, "It's like you're a leper. Nobody wants to come anywhere near you because they think the failure is contagious."[5]

Leprosy and the myths that surround it also remain a convenient weapon for those who want to demonize others. In 2003, the *New York Times* ran a story under the headline "Leprosy, a Synonym for a Stigma, Returns." The reporter wrote that more than seven thousand individuals in the United States had the disease, and that many were immigrants from "global leprosy hot spots, like Brazil, India, and the Caribbean." The story was only partly true. There were not seven thousand *existing* cases. Instead, seven thousand new cases had been reported over the previous *three decades* combined. Most of those patients had already been treated and cured. Still, the article quoted a doctor speculating that the thousands of cases identified were only "the ones we know about. . . . There are probably many, many more." The story made it appear as though the United States were on the verge of a terrifying outbreak.[6]

What's worse is that the article's error was picked up, repeated, and exaggerated by those who used it to rail against undocumented immigrants. Conservative writer Frosty Wooldridge incorrectly claimed that seven thousand cases of leprosy had entered the United States over a *three-year* period "on the backs of newcomers." Echoing nineteenth-century warnings about "leprous" Chinese laundry workers, Wooldridge added this ominous note: "Because illegal and legal immigrants are hired into food service, dish washing, cooking, hotels and day care—leprosy finds speedy access across the country." Nothing could be further from the truth, but the inaccurate information was repeated and spread by others, including Lou Dobbs on CNN, who said that, if anything, the seven-thousand figure was low. "The invasion of illegal aliens is threatening the health of many Americans," warned Dobbs.[7]

The threat of immigrants bringing leprosy into the country was again exaggerated in the 2018 debate over what to do about a "caravan" of people headed to the U.S. border from Central America. A former immigration agent claimed on Fox News that these immigrants were "coming in with diseases such as smallpox and leprosy and TB that are going to infect our people in the United States." President Trump got on the bandwagon a few weeks later. He did not specifically mention leprosy but said, without evidence, "People with tremendous medical difficulty and medical problems are pouring in, and in many cases it's contagious."[8] He made similar claims during his 2016 presidential campaign. Immigrants. Disease. Leprosy. As always, surefire dog whistles for stoking fear.

After Carville had closed and the patients were gone, it remained a monument to its unusual past. Some things have changed, for sure. Young Louisiana National Guardsmen greet visitors at the front gate. They can be seen in their camouflage uniforms and boots walking across the pastoral grounds and conducting drills with troubled teens who have come there to be straightened out. The plantation mansion still dominates the property. It stands gleaming and white along the now-paved river road, with its Corinthian columns gracing the second-floor balcony. Inside is an elegant dining room—where the original owner and his guests once partied for days—with a long, highly polished table beneath three glass chandeliers; the room is available for special events. Nearby, a one-story building that was once used for staff dining is now a museum, where the artifacts of Carville are carefully displayed and stored—a Mardi Gras float in the shape of an armadillo, medical equipment used to treat disabled limbs, photos of patient baseball games and shows, back copies of *The Star*, even the bronze bust that Tallulah Bankhead sent to an adoring Stanley Stein. Visitors drop by, one or two at a time, drawn by curiosity to what is still an out-of-the-way place. Many can't believe what they see.

Not far from the museum, the former infirmary has been renovated so that the rooms where Stein and so many other patients were treated and died can be used for conferences and guests. The recreation hall is used for gatherings, too, although the old patient post-office boxes remain empty and broken.

In many ways, Carville does not look much different than it did when hundreds of patients made it their home. The dorms and covered walkways remain standing, although they're dusty and deserted, with ripped screens flapping in the wind. Afternoon sunlight still pours through the windows and archways, casting a peaceful, even romantic, glow. Hundreds of birds, maybe thousands, still rest in the trees. Live oaks still line the front of the property, near the hole in the fence, which is now sealed off with a metal grate. Some of the trees are hundreds of years old and have lived through it all.

At a hospital in Baton Rouge, the National Hansen's Disease Program continues to treat patients from around the country and the world. In 2018, many came from the Marshall Islands, where the disease remains endemic. Doctors treat the patients' sores and disabilities and get them on the right medication, so they can return home. Special shoes are constructed for those who need them. Social workers and therapists are available to help the patients adjust to their new way of life, and the inevitable stigma.

———

On March 27, 2018, a half-dozen public health workers, a Catholic priest, and a visitor from Mexico followed a silver-gray casket up the steps of the Sacred Heart Chapel. The small party entered through the same front door that José Ramirez had so brazenly used years earlier.

The visitor was seventy-one-year-old Ramón Cabrera, son of Daniel Cabrera, one of the last-remaining Carville patients at St. Clare Manor nursing home in Baton Rouge. Daniel had died three days earlier at the age of ninety. Ramón's thin black hair was slicked back. He wore sunglasses and a navy blue striped polo shirt and jeans, looking more like a casual acquaintance of the deceased than a son about to bury his father.

Ramón had learned only a few months before that his father had had Hansen's disease and that this was why Daniel had been separated from the family for decades. When Ramón was a young child in Mexico, he was told that his father was dead. He soon learned that was not true, when Daniel shocked the family by showing up unannounced after he was initially released from Carville. Eventually, Daniel, a U.S. citizen, had a recurrence of Hansen's disease and returned to the hospital. Ramón got used to his father's being away, but had no idea where he was and why. They sometimes talked on the phone and Daniel periodically sent checks, but he never visited. Ramón thought his father was in the United States working to support the family.

Father and son were finally reunited in 2015, when a social worker with the National Hansen's Disease Program tracked Ramón down and told him that his father was an ailing patient at a nursing home in Baton Rouge. Even then, Daniel did not want his son to know why he was there. He had always been self-conscious about his appearance and his disease. When he was a younger patient at Carville, Daniel was often ridiculed by other patients for his awkward gait and tendency to fall—a symptom of neurological damage, doctors believed. Later, at the nursing home, Daniel would not go with the other patients on excursions to restaurants and elsewhere for fear of being laughed at. His skin was mottled, but he looked no different from many elderly men. In his room, Daniel had a photo of his younger self, taken around 1950, shortly before he was brought to Carville for the first time. His skin is smooth, almost translucent, his eyebrows thick and dark, his smile pleasant and assured. He said he never returned home when he finally could because he didn't want his family to see what had become of that handsome young man.[9]

Ramón learned the truth about his father, but his two brothers never did. One died as a child. The other was killed in a car crash as an adult. Ramón said that brother was an alcoholic, something he had always attributed to their father's absence. Still, Ramón was happy to be reunited with his father so he could be with him in his final days.[10]

Standing behind Cabrera's casket at the altar, the priest told the small group of mourners something they knew better than most, that Cabrera had not chosen the disease that brought him to Carville, so far from his home. Victims of leprosy may have been scorned by much of society, said the priest, but "this wonderful place became for these patients a place of mercy. Somebody cared enough to give them the love and care and dignity that they deserved as a fellow human being."

Cabrera's funeral was one of the last to be held at Carville. It was almost the end, both of a long, painful journey for a stigmatized group of people, and of a well-meaning but misguided effort to protect public health. Cabrera's body was laid to rest in the Carville cemetery near a pecan tree and alongside the graves of more than 750 other patients. Another 135 patients of the Louisiana Leper Home—including Clara Mertz, the woman who arrived under cover of night with that very first group—were buried in a nearby courtyard. They're identified on a plaque as they were known when they died, by their patient numbers and first name or initials. "No. 33 May." "No. 102 Hank." "No. 188 D. F." "No. 207 J. S." Anonymous, even in death.

Epilogue

———————

IN 2008, AFTER Harold Koll died, his son Matt—my husband—and I returned to Carville for a visit and to look at some of the artifacts stored at the museum. They included a voucher that Morris had signed to acknowledge the fifteen dollars he carried with him when he arrived from New York. Completely blind, his hands incapacitated, Morris had scrawled "X" next to his alias, Morris Krug, which was neatly written in script, presumably by a Daughter of Charity. It was one of the few signs Matt had that his grandfather had ever lived there.

From Carville, we took the half-hour drive to the small Jewish cemetery in Baton Rouge where Morris was buried. Much to our surprise, the gravestone was now stained with mildew, overgrown with weeds, and almost completely obscured from view. A sleeping bag and trash were scattered nearby, and an empty soda cup had been placed on top of a nearby headstone. This isolated corner of the cemetery had become someone's home.

We cleared away as much of the area as we could, but my husband decided then and there to have his grandfather's remains moved somewhere else. Like so many others with Hansen's disease, Morris Koll had been demeaned in life. He could at least be honored in death. As a veteran, Morris was eligible to be buried at Arlington Cemetery, where, coincidentally, President Taft, who was with him in the Philippines and New Haven, was also buried.

The process was set in motion to have Morris's remains exhumed, cremated, and brought back north. One of the biggest hurdles was that Morris had assumed so many identities as he moved from one stage of life to another. He was born Kolnitzky, although it was sometimes spelled Kolnitsky. After he returned from the Philippines, he legally changed his name to Koll, which he used until he was taken to Carville. There he became Morris Krug. The name on his tombstone—Kolnsky—was never correct, but it was the name he had used to enlist. Fortunately, the military patiently worked with Matt as he unraveled decades of paperwork discrepancies.

The military funeral was held on a sunny but cool December day in Arlington Cemetery, on an incline overlooking the nation's capital. Morris's cremated remains, along with those of his wife, Dora, were stored in small wooden boxes to be placed in the cemetery's columbarium. As family and friends sat under a canopy on an expanse of lawn, seven riflemen fired into the air, three times each. With the shots still echoing in the distance, a bugler slowly played "Taps," one soulful note after another. Six soldiers, wearing crisp white gloves, held the American flag outstretched over Morris's and Dora's remains and, with extraordinary precision, folded it into a thick, tight triangle. The officer in charge then turned to my husband, the next of kin, and, getting down on one knee, handed him the flag. "Sir, on behalf of the president of the United States, the United States Army, and a grateful nation, please accept this flag as a symbol of our appreciation for your loved one's honorable and faithful service," he said.

A volunteer—one of the Arlington Ladies, who attend every funeral there to ensure that no military member or veteran is ever buried alone—whispered to Matt how sorry she was for his loss and how Morris had been an inspiration to all. Hers were the sincere words of someone trying to console the bereaved, but it was a jarring moment for us. This was not a somber occasion at all. It was a joyous event. A soldier who had died almost eighty years earlier and fought in a battle more than a century ago was finally being honored. It was an incredible tribute to the value of life and a recognition that a man had died, and was incarcerated, because of a disease he contracted while serving his country.

The Arlington service was held in 2016, more than 120 years after the first patients had arrived at Carville, carrying with them the burden of centuries of ignorance and public disdain. So much progress has been made since that time. Still, when Matt requested his grandfather's medical records, he was assured by the clerk at the National Hansen's Disease Program in Baton Rouge that the documents would be mailed to him in a plain manila envelope. There would be no return address to reveal the sender. The family secret was safe.

Acknowledgments

I have always wanted to write a book, but it took the right topic and the help of countless others to turn that hope into what you now hold in your hands. My agent, Gail Ross, is the one who nudged me along, by saying at the right time, "I want you to write a book." She had a different one in mind, but that was all the encouragement I needed. She, along with Howard Yoon and Dara Kaye, helped me to reshape my ideas into a compelling story. I am grateful to Katie Henderson Adams, the Liveright editor who saw such promise in a book about leprosy. Her joy in the written word and in storytelling is an inspiration. She's since moved out on her own, but she left me in good hands. I'm thankful to editors Marie Pantojan and Dan Gerstle and the rest of the Liveright team, including Peter Miller, Gina Iaquinta, Haley Bracken, and Sarah Johnson, for doing the heavy lifting and guiding this project to completion. I am so fortunate that my first book is associated with such a stellar group.

I had no idea before I began researching the history of Carville how valuable good archives can be. The Daughters of Charity were meticulous chroniclers of their lives and work, and their archives in Emmitsburg, Maryland, are a gold mine of information. I knew that from the start, when one of my first discoveries was a 1935 entry in the sisters' annals—"Twelve patients have arrived in the past few days; four from New York, one a native of . . . Russia"—which marked the arrival of my husband's grandfather at the hospital. I took a photo and immediately texted it to my husband. "Look what I just found!" Thanks to Bonnie Weatherly and Scott Keefer for helping me find so much more. The LSU Libraries Special Collections were also invaluable, with their carefully preserved records of the Louisiana Leper Home. So, too, was the Louisiana Digital Library, which has stored online every edition of the patients' crusading newspaper, *The Star*, to which I must have referred hundreds of times. *The Star*, more than anything else, brings the history of Carville to life. I owe the greatest thanks, though, to Elizabeth Schexnyder, curator of the National Hansen's Disease Museum, who has painstakingly preserved the history of both this unique institution and the people who lived and worked there. Elizabeth knows almost everything there is to know about Carville, and I felt quite a sense of achievement those very few times I discovered a fact that was new to her. She was both incredibly generous with her time and patient with my endless requests and questions. Without her, there would be no book.

I am also thankful to the many people who were willing to share their personal stories and professional expertise with me. I realized early on that there were many others who were as eager as I was to tell the world about Carville. I had the good fortune to interview some of the last remaining patients at the Baton Rouge nursing home shortly before they died, including Simeon Peterson, Daniel Cabrera, and George Saldana. Other former patients—including José Ramirez, Mien Pham, and Francisco Sanchez—spent hours telling me their sometimes heart-wrenching personal stories. Family members of patients also willingly shared their memories and family lore. I'm especially grateful to Claire Manes and Gina DeRose Bell, whose relatives' writings greatly informed this book. Thanks, too, to Jack and Genie Dyer, Dolores Enriquez-Boehmer, Linda Williams, Ramón Cabrera, Cathy and Gerald Cousin, James Carville, Marcia Gaudet, Michelle Moran, John Parascandola, Nicole Lurie, and Magnus Vollset for their wonderful insights about Carville, Hansen's disease, and public health. Tom Adams of the Forty and Eight, which continues to publish *The Star* to this day, helped ensure that this story would be told.

A number of past and present employees of the National Hansen's Disease Program were extremely generous with their time and help. Thanks to David Scollard, Pamela Bartlett, Betsy Wilks, and Johanna Martinez. Government employees don't always get the credit they deserve for the work they do. I am forever grateful to Lila Davis, the U.S. Public Health Service employee who not only tracked down Morris Koll's burial site in Baton Rouge but cleaned his tombstone so it would shine brilliantly when his seventy-eight-year-old son saw his father's grave for the first time.

I also could not have done this book without the help of my bosses at NPR, especially Vickie Walton-James, who generously allowed me to take a year off from my day job to pursue this venture. I owe a great deal to many other colleagues who took time out of their busy lives to help. Marisa Peñaloza not only provided translations but, more important, told me that her son Diego was so fascinated when he heard the story of Carville that he went on the computer to learn everything he could about leprosy. He was my inspiration in moments of doubt. If a ten-year-old boy cared that much, this was a story that others would want to hear.

Wanting to tell a story is one thing. Writing it is another. I am indebted to Bonny Wolf, Jennifer Ludden, Luke Albee, and Steve Drummond, some of the best editors and most insightful readers around. They took my earliest drafts and helped turn them into something much more readable. Their enthusiasm for the project— "Hey, this is actually good!"—made me believe they weren't being so supportive just because they're my friends. Others, including June Beard, Beth Donovan, and Lynne Ganek, also helped me with their constant encouragement and interest in how I was doing. I am especially indebted to two of my oldest and dearest friends, both authors themselves, who guided me along this lengthy and sometimes grueling journey. Thank you so much, Joan Biskupic and Diane Kiesel. Along with Bonny, you were always there for me with the wisest advice, the perfect amount of sympathy, and your total confidence that I would do exactly what I set out to do. I will never forget your support.

The genesis of this book was my family. Thanks to Carol Sirkin Wood and Lenny Koll for providing insight into their grandfather's life, and especially to my sister-in-law Pearl Weiss, who was the first to discover that Morris Koll had been taken to Carville. None of this story would have been known had it not been for Valerie Reicheg, who encouraged her Uncle Harold to reveal the secret of his father's illness. Thank you, Valerie. And thank you, Harold, for listening to your niece.

My sons, Peter and David Koll, are the reason I wrote this book. This story is part of their legacy and I believe it's one of the things that's made them such socially responsible, hardworking young men. They care deeply about the world and their family (which joyfully gained Gina Holman during the course of my writing). They were extremely understanding when their mother was too distracted and fatigued these past two years to pay as much attention to them as they deserved. Peter was always available with his encouragement and wonderful food, and inspired me with his energetic approach to life. I owe a special thanks to David, who read not only my early drafts but every other version of the book. He was my toughest editor by far and used his screen-writing sensibility and skills to push his journalist mother to turn a bunch of facts into an interesting narrative. He is a gifted writer and editor. I am very grateful, and extremely proud.

Of course, my greatest—and lengthiest—thanks go to my wonderful husband, Matthew Koll. When I started this project, I began writing a list (seriously—it's sitting on my desk) of the many jobs he filled. He was my IT guy, legal adviser, business manager, PR consultant, web designer, barista, chef, personal trainer, mental health counselor, dog walker, spiritual adviser, research assistant—the list goes on and on. How anyone writes a book without such a supportive spouse is beyond me. True, this is partly his family's story, but Matt was much more patient, understanding, and encouraging than I had any right to expect. He gave up countless hours of his own time, and our time together, to see this project through. I love him, and our sons, dearly and forever.

Notes

Prologue

1 James Edgar Allen and John J. Reidy, *The Battle of Bayan and Other Battles* (Manila: E. C. McCullough & Co., 1903); Returns for the 27th Infantry, April 1902–December 1903, National Archives Microfilm Publication M665, roll 268 (Washington, DC: National Archives Building [NAB]); Robert A. Fulton, "A Brief History of America and the Moros, 1899–1920," http://www.morolandhistory.com, 8–9.

2 Daniel Hannefin, DC, "The Daughters of Charity at Carville: 1896–1981," *Vincentian Heritage Journal*, 2, no. 1 (1981), 63–64; Sister Ursula Bertschy, DC, "A History of the United States Leper Colony" (master's thesis, DePaul University, 1949), 112.

3 Author interview with Daniel Cabrera, Baton Rouge, LA, May 24, 2016.

4 If you search online for synonyms for *pariah*, one of the first words that comes up is *leper*.

5 Based on author's numerous conversations with Harold Koll.

Chapter 1: Exile

1 "Cruel Neglect: How the City Government Cares for Its Grievously Afflicted," *Daily Picayune*, February 18, 1893.

2 "Mardi Gras: A Grand Celebration of the Carnival for the Twenty-First Time," *Daily Picayune*, February 15, 1893.

3 Erin Blakemore, "The Grisly Story of America's Largest Lynching,"

"History Stories," History, October 25, 2017, http://www.history.com
.news/the-grisly-story-of-americas-largest-lynching.
4 History of New Orleans, the port, and epidemics based on numerous
   sources, including Urma Engineer Willoughby, *Yellow Fever, Race and
   Ecology in Nineteenth-Century New Orleans* (Baton Rouge: Louisiana State
   University Press, 2017); Harold Sinclair, *The Port of New Orleans* (Garden
   City, NY: Doubleday, Doran, 1942); Orleans Parish Medical Society,
   The Daily Picayune: A Year in Review, 1878, http://www.opms.org/images/
   stories/OPMS-History-Profile.pdf.
5 Zachary Gussow, *Leprosy, Racism and Public Health* (Boulder: Westview
   Press, 1989), 39.
6 "Leprosy in New Orleans," *Daily Picayune*, March 19, 1892.
7 John Smith Kendall, "How I Started a Hospital," *The Fossil*, October 1959,
   National Library of Medicine (NLM), Public Health Service Hospitals
   Historical Collection 1895–1982 (PHSHHC), MS C 471, Box 11, Folder 5.
8 "What Led to Founding the Carville Hospital: A Little Known Chapter,"
   Star, 14, no. 3, November–December 1954.
9 "Cruel Neglect."
10 "Louisiana Leper Board Organized," *New York Times*, September 2,
   1894.
11 Isadore Dyer, "The History of the Louisiana Leper Home," *New Orleans
   Medical and Surgical Journal*, 54 (May 1902), 714.
12 Gussow, *Leprosy, Racism, and Public Health*, 44.
13 Gussow, 48, 53.
14 Gussow, 128.
15 "White Laundrymen Combine to Boycott the St. Louis Patrons of
   Chinese Rivals," *Daily Picayune*, July 17, 1892.
16 Gussow, *Leprosy, Racism, and Public Health*, 56.
17 Gussow, 105.
18 "A Leprosy Case," *Daily Picayune*, August 15, 1891.
19 "Lepers and Leprosy," *Daily Picayune*, May 26, 1893.
20 "A Disgrace to the City," *Daily Picayune*, November 15, 1893.
21 *Archives of Dermatology and Syphilology*, vol. 2 (Chicago: American Medical
   Association, 1920), 757.
22 *Who's Who in Louisiana and Mississippi*, published by the *Times-Picayune*,
   July 1918, 77.
23 Henry Cohen, "Settlement of the Jews in Texas," *Publications of the
   American Jewish Historical Society*, no. 2 (1894), 139–56.
24 Author interviews with Dyer's grandchildren, Jack and Genie Dyer,
   New Orleans, LA, March 19, 2018; and family records. Almost a
   hundred years after her grandfather's death, Genie Dyer still kept a copy
   of "Each Day" taped by her bedside.
25 Dyer, "The History," 716.

26 "The Leper Board Ready for Business," *Daily Picayune*, September 11, 1894.

27 "The Leper Hospital Again," *Daily Picayune*, November 10, 1894.

28 "Gentilly Road Will Have No Lepers," *Daily Picayune*, November 17, 1894.

29 Letter from Gaston Mesier to Dr. Henry J. Scherck, 1894, General Correspondence, Folder 1, Louisiana Leper Home Records (LLHR), Mss. 2515, Louisiana and Lower Mississippi Valley Collections, LSU Libraries, Baton Rouge, LA.

30 Kendall, "How I Started a Hospital."

31 "The Leper Board Begins Its Work; Seven Sufferers Quietly Removed from the Local Hospital," *Daily Picayune*, December 2, 1894.

32 "Proud Ante-Bellum Mansion Enacts Role in Medical Drama," *Star*, 14, no. 3 (November–December 1954).

33 "L. A. Carville from Carville, La," *Star*, 14, no. 3 (November–December 1954).

Chapter 2: God versus Germs

1 Lev. 13:45–46.

2 Silatham Sermrittirong and W. H. van Brakel, "Stigma in Leprosy: Concepts, Causes and Determinants," *Leprosy Review*, 85, no. 1 (2014), 41; Rod Edmond, *Leprosy and Empire: A Medical and Cultural History* (Cambridge: Cambridge University Press, 2006), 9.

3 Frederick C. Lendrum, "The Name 'Leprosy,'" *American Journal of Tropical Medicine and Hygiene*, 1, no. 6 (November 1952).

4 Nick Farrell, Oral History, September 12, 1996, National Hansen's Disease Museum (NHDM), Acct. 21014, Carville, LA.

5 Saul Nathaniel Brody, *The Disease of the Soul: Leprosy in Medieval Literature* (Ithaca: Cornell University Press, 1974), 51.

6 Brody, *The Disease of the Soul*, 66–68.

7 Brody, 69.

8 Brody, 103.

9 Brody, 41.

10 Brody, 100.

11 Brody, 87; Carole Rawcliffe, "The Form and Function of Medieval Hospitals" (lecture, Grisham College, London, August 31, 2011).

12 Zachary Gussow and George S. Tracy, "The Use of Archival Materials in the Analysis and Interpretation of Field Data: A Case Study in the Institutionalization of the Myth of Leprosy as 'Leper,'" *American Anthropologist*, New Series, 73, no. 3 (June 1971), 695–709.

13 Lew Wallace, *Ben-Hur: A Tale of the Christ* (1880; repr., Blacksburg, VA: Wilder Publications, 2011), 387.

14 Zachary Gussow, *Leprosy, Racism, and Public Health: Social Policy in Chronic Disease Control* (Boulder: Westview Press, 1989), 205.

15 Gussow, *Leprosy, Racism, and Public Health*, 72.

16 Danielssen and Boeck called the two forms of the disease by different names from those used today. They called tuberculoid leprosy "anesthetic" and lepromatous leprosy "tubercular." Other forms of leprosy have since been identified, including "mixed" or "borderline," which combines symptoms of the other two.

17 Hansen married Stephanie Danielssen in 1873. She died soon after from tuberculosis.

18 Tony Gould, *A Disease Apart: Leprosy in the Modern World* (New York: St. Martin's Press, 2005), 44.

19 Th. M. Vogelsang, "Leprosy in Norway," *Medical History*, 9, no. 1 (1965), 33.

20 Yngve Nedrebø, ed., *Leprosy* (Bergen: The Leprosy Archives of Bergen), 37.

21 Andrzej Grzybowski, Guido Kluxen, and Klaudia Poltorak, "Gerhard Henrik Armauer Hansen (1841–1912)—100 Years Anniversary Tribute," *Acta Ophthalmologica*, 92 (2014), 296–300.

22 Th. M. Vogelsang, "A Serious Sentence Passed against the Discoverer of the Leprosy Bacillus (Gerhard Armauer Hansen), in 1880," *Medical History*, 7, no. 2 (1963), 182–86; Michael F. Marmor, "The Ophthalmic Trials of G. H. A. Hansen," *Survey of Ophthalmology*, 7, no. 3 (May–June 2002), 275–87. Hansen might have been influenced by his reported dislike of women's emancipation. He also did not believe that women should be doctors. Almost a century later a female doctor in the United States would succeed where he had failed, becoming the first scientist to infect an animal (an armadillo) with leprosy.

23 Vogelsang, "A Serious Sentence Passed," 185.

24 Jo Robertson, "The Leprosy-Affected Body as a Commodity: Autonomy and Compassion," in *The Body Divided: Human Beings and Human 'Material' in Modern Medical History*, ed. Sarah Ferber and Sally Wilde (Surrey, UK: Ashgate, 2011), 131.

25 Gould, *A Disease Apart*, 51.

26 Gussow, *Leprosy, Racism, and Public Health*, 79.

Chapter 3: Rescue Mission

1 "The Leper Board Begins Its Work: Seven Sufferers Quietly Removed from the Local Hospital," *Daily Picayune*, December 2, 1894.

2 "The Lepers' Home," *Catholic Tribune*, June 26, 1897.

3 "The Lepers," *Daily Picayune*, December 22, 1894.

4 Isadore Dyer, "The History of the Louisiana Leper Home," *New Orleans Medical and Surgical Journal*, 54 (May 1902), 718.

5 "The Leper Board: Refuses to Remove the Hospital from Its Present Site," *Daily Picayune*, December 28, 1894.

6 "The Care of the Lepers," *Daily Picayune*, December 29, 1894.

7 Letter dated January 9, 1895, from Iberville police jury to Isadore Dyer, and board's February 6 response, General Correspondence, Folder 1, LLHR.

8 "The Leper Board: Decides to Stand upon Its Rights under the Law," *Daily Picayune*, January 9, 1895.

9 "Gathering in the Wandering Lepers," *Daily Picayune*, January 19, 1895.

10 Dyer, "The History," 721.

11 "Proclamation," *Daily Picayune*, January 27, 1895.

12 "The Leper Hospital Made a Real Home: The Board of Control Deems the Disease Contagious, and Urges the Proper Authorities to Take Steps," *Daily Picayune*, May 8, 1895.

13 Correspondence from L. A. Wailes to the Board of Control, May–September 1895, General Correspondence, Folders 5–6, LLHR.

14 "The Leper Board Wants the Sisters," *Daily Picayune*, September 4, 1895; "Sisters of Charity Will Care for Lepers," *Daily Picayune*, November 25, 1895.

15 Letter from Sister Agnes Slavin to Mother Mariana Flynn, February 29, 1896, quoted in Sr. Hilary Ross, "Leprosarium, Carville, LA, 1894–1958," RG 11-2-2 Carville, LA—Hansen's Disease Center, Archives of the Daughters of Charity (DOC), Province of St. Louise, Emmitsburg, MD, 28.

16 Sister Ursula Bertschy, DC, "A History of the United States Leper Colony" (master's thesis, DePaul University, 1949), 71.

17 "Four Women on a Heroic Mission," *Daily Picayune*, April 17, 1896.

18 "The Sisters at the Leper Camp Now," *Daily Picayune*, April 23, 1896.

19 Letter from Sister Beatrice to Sister Josephine, May 10, 1896, quoted in Ross, "Leprosarium."

20 "The Colorful Characters of Carville," *Star*, 61, nos. 1–4 (January–December 2002).

21 Ross, "Leprosarium," 30.

22 Ross, 43.

23 Ross, 57.

24 Ross, 44–46.

25 Ross, 34.

26 Bertschy, "A History," 108.

27 Julia Elwood, ed., *With Love in Their Hearts: The Daughters of Charity of St. Vincent De Paul, 1896–1996* (Washington, DC: U.S. Public Health Service, 1996), 23–24.

28 "A Visit Paid to the Leper Land," *Daily Picayune*, January 24, 1897.

29 "Three Members of the Leper Board Send in Resignations and Their Successors Were Chosen," *Daily Picayune*, July 9, 1896.

30 "No One Wants the Lepers," *New York Sun*, July 19, 1896.

31 Daniel Hannefin, DC, "The Daughters of Charity at Carville: 1896–1981," *Vincentian Heritage Journal*, 2, no. 1 (1981): 58.

32 Letter from Sister Beatrice to Mother Mariana, August 16, 1896, Daughters of Charity Annals, vols. 1 and 2, 1894–1921, 16767, NHDM.

33 Letter from Sister Beatrice to M. D. Lagan, June 13, 1897, General Correspondence, Folder 10, LLHR.

34 Based on numerous letters from Sister Beatrice to the Board of Control, 1898–1900, General Correspondence, Folder 10, LLHR; Ross, "Leprosarium," 33.

35 Dyer, "The History," 722.

36 "Report of the Secretaries of the International Leprosy Conference, Berlin, 1897," quoted in *Leprosy in the United States, U.S. Senate Committee on Public Health and National Quarantine*, S. Doc. 269, 57th Cong., 1st session (March 24, 1902), 43.

37 Bi-annual Report of the Board of Control of the Leper Home of the State of Louisiana, 1898.

38 "Leper Home Not Wanted in Jefferson Parish," *Daily Picayune*, May 11, 1901.

39 "The Leper Hospital," *Daily Picayune*, May 11, 1901.

40 "Leper Buildings Fired," *Times-Democrat*, May 24, 1901.

41 "Jefferson Uses the Torch of Defiance," *Daily Picayune*, May 24, 1901.

42 "Sister Beatrice of the Lepers," RG 10-2 Individual Sisters—Sr. Beatrice Hart, DOC.

43 Letter from Sister Beatrice to Albert Phelps of the Louisiana Leper Home Board of Control, August 4, 1901, General Correspondence, Folder 19, LLHR.

Chapter 4: Rebellion

1 James R. Arnold, *The Moro War: How America Battled a Muslim Insurgency in the Philippine Jungle, 1902–1913* (New York: Bloomsbury Press, 2011), 27.

2 Arnold, *The Moro War*, 30–31.

3 "Hearts and Minds in Mindanao," *Military History*, September 28, 2017.

4 James Herman Pruitt II, "Leonard Wood and the American Empire" (PhD diss., Texas A&M University, 2011).

5 Victor G. Heiser, "Leprosy in the Philippine Islands," *Public Health Reports*, 24, no. 33 (August 13, 1909): 1155–1159.

6 Zachary Gussow, *Leprosy, Racism, and Public Health: Social Policy in Chronic Disease Control* (Boulder: Westview Press, 1989), 135.

7 "Future Disposition of Leper Colony," *San Francisco Call*, April 21, 1899.

8 Michelle T. Moran, *Colonizing Leprosy: Imperialism and the Politics of Public Health in the United States* (Chapel Hill: University of North Carolina Press, 2007), 25.

9 *Leprosy in the United States, U.S. Senate Committee on Public Health and National Quarantine*, S. Doc. 269, 57th Cong., 1st session (March 24, 1902), 8.

10 *Leprosy in the United States*, 71.

11 *Leprosy in the United States*, 82.

12 *Leprosy in the United States*, 10.

13 Philip A. Kalisch, "Lepers, Anachronisms, and the Progressives: A Study in Stigma, 1889–1920," *Louisiana Studies*, 12 (Fall 1973): 506.

14 Kalisch, "Lepers, Anachronisms," 505.

15 Moran, *Colonizing Leprosy*, 36.

16 Joint Resolution 8, Acts of the Legislative Assembly of the Territory of New Mexico, 35th and 36th Sessions. Copy in Stanley Stein archives, 196881, NHDM.

17 Gussow, *Leprosy, Racism, and Public Health*, 139.

18 Moran, *Colonizing Leprosy*, 32–38.

19 Letter from Sister Benedicta to Albert Phelps, April 29, 1902, General Correspondence, Folder 20, LLHR.

20 "The Leper Board Begins Its Work: Seven Sufferers Quietly Removed from the Local Hospital," *Daily Picayune*, December 2, 1894.

21 Daniel Hannefin, DC, "The Daughters of Charity at Carville: 1896–1981," *Vincentian Heritage Journal*, 2, no. 1 (1981): 62.

22 Letter from Sister Benedicta to Mother Margaret O'Keefe, July 12, 1902, RG 11-2, DOC.

23 *Bi-annual Report of the Board of Control for the Leper Home of the State of Louisiana*, 1902, 30.

24 *Bi-annual Report of the Board of Control*, 23.

25 Letter from Sister Benedicta to Mother Margaret, July 12, 1902, RG 11-2, DOC.

26 *Bi-annual Report of the Board of Control*, 33–35.

27 Isadore Dyer, "The History of the Louisiana Leper Home," *New Orleans Medical and Surgical Journal*, 54 (May 1902): 732.

28 Letter from Sister Benedicta to Albert Phelps, September 6, 1902, General Correspondence, Folder 21, LLHR.

29 Letter from W. J. Abrams to Albert Phelps, September 7, 1902, General Correspondence, Folder 21, LLHR.

30 Letter from Sister Benedicta to board secretary John Pollock, May 23, 1906, General Correspondence, Folder 31, LLHR.

31 Letter from Sister Benedicta to John Pollock, May 26, 1906, General Correspondence, Folder 31, LLHR.

32 *Biennial Report of the Board of Control for the Leper Home of the State of Louisiana*, 1906, 9.

33 Letter to Leper Home Board of Control from Iberville residents, November 10, 1906, General Correspondence, Folder 34, LLHR.

34 Letter from Sister Benedicta to Leper Home Board of Control, March 13, 1905, General Correspondence, Folder 26, LLHR.
35 Letter from Sister Benedicta to Leper Home Board, November 12, 1907, General Correspondence, Folder 38, LLHR.
36 Letter from Leper Home Board Secretary Pollock to patients, November 18, 1907, General Correspondence, Folder 38, LLHR.
37 Letter to the Leper Home Board from the Patients' Committee, July 1, 1907, General Correspondence, Folder 36, LLHR.
38 Letter to the Leper Home Board from the Patients' Committee, July 24, 1907, General Correspondence, Folder 36, LLHR.
39 *Biennial Report of the Board of Control for the Leper Home of the State of Louisiana*, 1914.
40 Kalisch, "Lepers, Anachronisms," 508.

Chapter 5: "What Have I Got, Doctor—Leprosy?"

1 John Early, *Angel—Devil—Brute—Man* (self-published memoir, date unknown, estimated 1928). Copy provided to author by Early's great-granddaughter, Gina DeRose Bell.
2 Philip A. Kalisch, "The Strange Case of John Early: A Study of the Stigma of Leprosy," *International Journal of Leprosy*, 40, no. 3 (1972): 291–305.
3 "Leper in Washington," *Baltimore Sun*, August 24, 1908.
4 "Leprosy in the District," *Sunday Star*, August 23, 1908.
5 "Medical Men Deprecate Danger of Leprosy," *Washington Times*, August 25, 1908.
6 "In Effort to See Leper Early Curious Throngs Dodge Guards," *Washington Times*, September 5, 1908.
7 Early, *Angel—Devil*, 129–35.
8 Izola Forrester, "The Strange Case of John Early," *Munsey's Magazine*, 41, no. 6, September 1909, 773–81.
9 "Leper's Pension Comes To-Morrow," *Washington Herald*, September 6, 1908.
10 "A Woman Would Chloroform Lepers," *Albuquerque Citizen*, September 5, 1908.
11 "Woman Leper Dies in County Hospital: Tragic and Pitiable End of Brave Soldier's Widow," *Wichita Daily Eagle*, December 3, 1908.
12 *Care and Treatment of Persons Afflicted with Leprosy, U.S. Senate Committee on Public Health and National Quarantine*, S. Rept. 306, 64th Cong. 1st session (March 25, 1916), 82–85 (testimony of Dr. John S. Fulton, secretary of the State Board of Health of Maryland).
13 "Leper on Detour," *Washington Post*, July 22, 1906.
14 "Leper Is Turned Back to South by Authorities," *Philadelphia Inquirer*, July 23, 1906.

15 "Back to His Box Car: Leper Alarmed Residents by Taking a Little Walk," *Baltimore Sun*, July 24, 1906.

16 "Syrian Leper Safe," *Cumberland Evening News*, October 10, 1906.

17 "Leper's Car Destroyed," *Democratic Advocate*, September 7, 1906.

18 "Cowards Made by Science," *Washington Post*, August 4, 1906.

19 John S. Fulton, ed.,"The Syrian Leper, George Rashid," *Maryland Medical Journal, Medicine and Surgery*, 29 (August 1906): 322–23.

20 "Can't Deport the Leper," *Baltimore Sun*, August 9, 1906.

21 Isadore Dyer, "The Sociological Aspects of Leprosy and the Question of Segregation" (paper presented to the New York Academy of Medicine, December 29, 1910), reprinted in *Journal of Cutaneous Diseases, Including Syphilis*, 29 (1911).

22 "Leprosy and Twentieth Century Civilization," *Medical Times*, 38 (February 1910): 51–52.

23 Kalisch, "The Strange Case of John Early," 295.

24 "Early Off at Last: Goes in Baggage Car," *Evening Star*, July 4, 1909.

25 "Early Free from Leprosy," *New York Times*, July 5, 1909.

26 "Personal and Impersonal," *Brooklyn Daily Eagle*, July 6, 1909.

27 "Hansen Says Early Was Leper," *Evening Star*, September 25, 1909.

28 "Problem on Hand: District Wrestling with Case of John Early," *Evening Star*, December 3, 1909.

29 "The Strange Case of John R. Early," *Washington Times*, December 4, 1909.

30 Early, *Angel—Devil*, 184–86.

31 "Leper's Presence Stirs Neighbors: Must Go, They Say," *Oregon Daily Journal*, February 2, 1912.

32 Early, *Angel—Devil*, 189.

33 Kalisch, "The Strange Case of John Early," 297.

34 "'I Lied,' Says Former Wife of Early," *Tacoma Times*, July 10, 1913.

35 Early, *Angel—Devil*, 196–97.

Chapter 6: Finding a Home

1 "Welcome for Early: Alleged Leper Brushes through Crowd," *New York Tribune*, July 5, 1909.

2 John Early, *Angel—Devil—Brute—Man* (self-published memoir, date unknown, estimated 1928), 197.

3 "Early Proud of Trip Here: Leper, Now Resigned, Tells How He Met Noted People," *Washington Herald*, June 4, 1914.

4 "Leper Early Is Caught Here by Health Officials," *Washington Times*, June 2, 1914.

5 "Early, the Leper, a Prisoner Here," *Evening Star*, June 2, 1914.

6 "Early Proud of Trip Here," *Washington Herald*, June 4, 1914.

7 "Case of John Early," *Washington Times*, June 4, 1914.

8   Philip A. Kalisch, "The Strange Case of John Early: A Study of the Stigma of Leprosy," *International Journal of Leprosy*, 40, no. 3 (1972): 298.

9   Transactions of the Section on Dermatology, American Medical Association, at the 65th Annual Session (June 23–26, 1914), 34–51.

10 "Burning Lepers in China," *Missionary Review of the World*, 36 (April 1913): 306.

11 Philip A. Kalisch, "Lepers, Anachronisms, and the Progressives: A Study in Stigma, 1889–1920," *Louisiana Studies*, 12 (Fall 1973): 525.

12 Michelle T. Moran, *Colonizing Leprosy: Imperialism and the Politics of Public Health in the United States* (Chapel Hill: University of North Carolina Press, 2007), 40.

13 *Care and Treatment of Persons Afflicted with Leprosy, U.S. Senate Committee on Public Health and National Quarantine*, S. Rept. 306, 64th Cong. 1st session (March 25, 1916), 81 (testimony of Dr. John S. Fulton, secretary of the State Board of Health of Maryland).

14 *Care and Treatment*, 146.

15 *Care and Treatment*, 13–38.

16 Stanley Stein, *Alone No Longer: The Story of a Man Who Refused to Be One of the Living Dead*, with Lawrence G. Blochman (New York: Funk and Wagnalls, 1963; repr., Star, 1974), 98.

17 Kalisch, "Lepers, Anachronisms," 517.

18 Kalisch, 519.

19 Victor Heiser, *An American Doctor's Odyssey: Adventures in Forty-Five Countries* (New York: W. W. Norton, 1936), 256.

20 Letter from Sister Benedicta to Oscar Dowling, president of the Louisiana Board of Health, June 11, 1919, Daughters of Charity Annals, vols. 1 and 2, 1894–1921, 16767, NHDM.

21 Early, *Angel—Devil*, 201–3.

22 Early, 204.

23 Early, 206.

24 "John Early, Leper, Again Flees from Prison Home," *Washington Times*, September 16, 1918.

25 *Eleventh Biennial Report of the Board of Control for the Leper Home of the State of Louisiana*, 1916, 26.

26 *Twelfth Biennial Report of the Board of Control for the Leper Home of the State of Louisiana*, 1918, 19.

27 Daniel Hannefin, DC, "The Daughters of Charity at Carville: 1896–1981," *Vincentian Heritage Journal*, 2, no. 1 (1981): 69.

28 Early, *Angel—Devil*, 209.

29 "U.S. Officials Unearth Secret Plan for Big Parade of Lepers in Capital," *Washington Times*, April 25, 1920.

30 "U.S. to Frustrate Escape of Lepers: Public Health Service Takes Precautions to Guard against Threatened Invasion," *Washington Times*, April 26, 1920.

31 "Daring Chief of Lepers Planning Capital Parade: Washington Gasps at Menace of Plot Uncovered There Recently," *Wichita Daily Eagle*, May 4, 1920.

Chapter 7: Ripped Apart

1 The Landry family story is based on personal interviews with Edmond Landry's granddaughter, Claire Manes, and her book, *Out of the Shadow of Leprosy* (Jackson: University Press of Mississippi, 2013), as well as on letters written by Norbert and Edmond Landry while they were patients at Carville.

2 *Eleventh Biennial Report of the Board of Control for the Leper Home of the State of Louisiana*, 1916, 17.

3 *Biennial Report of the Board of Control for the Leper Home of the State of Louisiana*, 1920, 17.

4 Letter from Norbert Landry to Edmond Landry, August 8, 1919, quoted in Manes, *Out of the Shadow*, 147–48.

5 Letter from Norbert to Edmond, March 10, 1921, in Manes, 166–68.

6 Manes, 166–68.

7 Marcia Gaudet, *Carville: Remembering Leprosy in America* (Jackson: University Press of Mississippi, 2004), 175.

8 A fourth child, Ruth, died from the flu in 1911 at the age of two.

9 Koll's account is from an interview he conducted with health officials at Carville while he was a patient there from 1935 to 1938, personal medical records, National Hansen's Disease Program, Baton Rouge, LA.

10 Letter from Norbert to Edmond, December 18, 1919, in Manes, *Out of the Shadow*, 157.

11 Entry dated January 12, 1936, in Daughters of Charity Annals 1930–1939, vol. 4, 16769, and entry dated April 3, 1942, in Annals 1940–1949, vol. 5, 16770, NHDM.

12 "Increase of Leprosy Danger to Public Health: Congress to Be Asked for Hospitals," *Bridgeport Telegram*, June 19, 1922.

13 "15 Lepers Are in St. Louis for Day on Way South," *St. Louis Post Dispatch*, March 17, 1922.

14 Gaudet, *Carville*, 41–43.

15 Letter from Edmond to Claire, April 28, 1927, in Manes, *Out of the Shadow*, 85–86.

16 Gaudet, *Carville*, 181.

17 "Mother Relies on Prayer to Save 2 Schoolboy Lepers," *New York Daily News*, June 26, 1925. One of the boys died ten years later from tuberculosis. His brother was released and went back home to live with their mother, according to Sr. Hilary Ross.

18 Gaudet, *Carville*, 46.

19 "Carville's Buddy," *Star*, 8, no. 5 (January 1949).

20 Author interview with Oscar Dempster's niece and her husband, Cathy and Gerald Cousin, Darrow, LA, December 5, 2018.

21 Gaudet, *Carville*, 175.

22 Gaudet, 176.

23 Betty Martin, *Miracle at Carville*, edited by Evelyn Wells (New York: Doubleday, 1951), 15.

Chapter 8: "Nun Nurses"

1 From account written by Sister Hilary Ross, RG 10-2 Individual Sisters—Sr. Hilary Ross, DOC.

2 Letter to the Ross family from Sister Mary Moran, December 12, 1982, RG 10-2 Individual Sisters—Sr. Hilary Ross, DOC.

3 Cynthia Gould, "Sister Hilary Ross and Carville: Her 37 Year Struggle against Hansen's Disease" (master's thesis, University of New Orleans, 1989), repr., *Star*, 50, no. 5 (May–June 1991) and no. 6 (July–August 1991).

4 From account written by Sister Hilary Ross, RG 10-2 Individual Sisters—Sr. Hilary Ross, DOC.

5 Speech by Dr. William Meyer at retirement ceremony for Sister Hilary Ross at Carville, RG 10-2 Individual Sisters—Sr. Hilary Ross, DOC.

6 Cynthia Gould, "Sister Hilary Ross," *Star*, 50, no. 5.

7 John Parascandola, "Chaulmoogra Oil and the Treatment of Leprosy," *Pharmacy in History*, 45, no. 2 (2003): 47–57.

8 Philip A. Kalisch, "Lepers, Anachronisms, and the Progressives: A Study in Stigma, 1889–1920," *Louisiana Studies*, 12 (Fall 1973): 523.

9 Stanley Stein, *Alone No Longer: The Story of a Man Who Refused to Be One of the Living Dead*, with Lawrence G. Blochman (New York: Funk and Wagnalls, 1963; repr., Star, 1974), 56.

10 History of the St. Louise Province, by Sr. Vincentine, RG 10-2 Individual Sisters—Sr. Catherine Sullivan, DOC.

11 "Sixty-Four," *Star*, 14, no. 3 (November–December, 1954).

12 "Lilies Bring Memories," *Star*, 5, no. 10 (June 1946).

13 From 1961 taped interview of Sister Catherine Sullivan, RG 11-2, DOC.

14 "Here and There—The Cornette," *Bulletin of the Holy Agony*, January–February–March 1946, RG 10-2 Individual Sisters—Sr. Catherine Sullivan, DOC.

15 Stein, *Alone No Longer*, 184.

16 John Early, *Angel—Devil—Brute—Man* (self-published memoir, date unknown, estimated 1928), 233.

17 Tony Gould, *A Disease Apart: Leprosy in the Modern World* (New York: St. Martin's Press, 2005), 207.

18 Letter to U.S. surgeon general from John McMullen, April 14, 1926, RG 90, Box 479, Folder 1850-95 (1934–35), NACP.

19 Stein, *Alone No Longer*, 61.

20 Patient petition dated August 28, 1924, to retain the sisters and patient testimony during Public Health Service investigation of conditions at Carville, May 24–27, 1926, RG 90, Box 479, Folder 1850-95, (1923–27), NACP.
21 Patient petition opposing firing of Protestant chaplain, May 20, 1926, RG 90, Box 479, Folder 1850-95 (1934–35).
22 Letter from McMullen to U.S. surgeon general Hugh S. Cumming, April 1, 1929, RG 90, Box 479, Folder 1850-95 (1928–33).
23 Inspection report from William Terriberry to U.S. surgeon general, January 10, 1935, RG 90, Box 479, Folder 1850-95 (1934–35).

Chapter 9: Jail Within a Jail

1 Letter from O. E. Denney to U.S. surgeon general, August 24, 1925, RG 90, Box 476, Folder 1205, NACP.
2 Stanley Stein, *Alone No Longer: The Story of a Man Who Refused to Be One of the Living Dead*, with Lawrence G. Blochman (New York: Funk and Wagnalls, 1963; repr., Star, 1974), 101.
3 O. E. Denney, "The National Leper Home (Marine Hospital No. 66)," *Public Health Reports*, 41, no. 46 (November 12, 1926): 2593–97.
4 O. E. Denney, "The Leprosy Problem in the United States," *Public Health Reports*, 41, no. 20 (May 14, 1926): 923–29.
5 Zachary Gussow, *Leprosy, Racism, and Public Health: Social Policy in Chronic Disease Control* (Boulder: Westview Press, 1989), 248–49.
6 Denney, "The Leprosy Problem in the United States."
7 Michelle T. Moran, *Colonizing Leprosy: Imperialism and the Politics of Public Health in the United States* (Chapel Hill: University of North Carolina Press, 2007), 99.
8 On March 13, 1940, the Daughters of Charity made this entry in their annals: "Charley Woo (the lost chinaman, as he has been called here) died to-day after receiving Baptism. He was admitted March 29, 1922, and has spent all these years in our jail, a raving maniac. His history was blank. We could never find out anything about him, except that he was admitted from a California hospital and called himself Charley Woo." Even though the sisters wrote that Woo came from a California hospital, it's likely that he was the same man who came with Hazel Deuser from St. Louis, where he had been confined at a hospital for more than fifteen years. In any event, Woo spent eighteen years in the Carville jail. Daughters of Charity Annals, 1940–1949, vol. 5, 16770, NHDM.
9 Letter from Denney to U.S. surgeon general, September 6, 1927, RG 90, Box 474, Folder 0245 (1925–27), NACP.
10 Letter from Denney to the assistant surgeon general, September 16, 1925, RG 90, Box 474, Folder 0245 (1925–27), NACP.
11 Philip A. Kalisch, "The Strange Case of John Early: A Study of the

Stigma of Leprosy," *International Journal of Leprosy*, 40, no. 3 (1972): 300.

12 John Early, *Angel—Devil—Brute—Man* (self-published memoir, date unknown, estimated 1928), 220.

13 "Camping Leper Having Fun as State Worries," *Asheville Citizen-Times*, April 21, 1927.

14 "Federal Posse Nabs Early in Mountain Hut," *Asheville Citizen-Times*, August 29, 1927.

15 Early, *Angel—Devil*, 237.

16 He is referred to in some accounts as Edward Peyton but is buried at Carville under the name of Edward Payton.

17 "Negro Leper Pleads Guilty, Given 10 Years," *Alexandria Daily Town Talk*, November 14, 1927.

18 "Case against Beaurepaire, Leper, Charged with Murder of Wife, Recalled," *Alexandria Daily Town Talk*, August 27, 1927.

19 Early, *Angel—Devil*, 238.

20 "Famous Leper, John Early Will Go Free, Cured," *Binghamton Press*, November 19, 1928.

Chapter 10: The Hole in the Fence

1 Stanley Stein, *Alone No Longer: The Story of a Man Who Refused to Be One of the Living Dead*, with Lawrence G. Blochman (New York: Funk and Wagnalls, 1963; repr., Star, 1974), 46.

2 Stein, *Alone No Longer*, 12.

3 Stein, 15.

4 Stein, 21.

5 Stein, 31.

6 Stein, 36.

7 Stein, 50.

8 Stein, 58.

9 Stein, 8–9.

10 Stein, 47.

11 Madeleine Pierron Patrick, "The Secret People: Patriotism, the Press, and Civil Rights in the National Leprosarium" (master's thesis, University of Georgia, 2013), 38.

12 Stein, *Alone No Longer*, 61.

13 Stein, 83.

14 Minstrel shows at the time generally had white performers appearing in blackface, and Carville was no exception.

15 Stein, *Alone No Longer*, 55.

16 Stein, 71.

17 Stein, 80.

18 "Frank Nesom: Patients' Pal," *Star*, 38, no. 1 (September–October 1978).

19 Sam H. Jones, "The Strangest Post in the World," *American Legion Monthly*, 19, no. 2 (August 1935), 18.

20 Stein, *Alone No Longer*, 118–19.

21 Stein, 124.

22 Stein, 146.

23 "Looking out from Within," *Sixty-Six Star*, 2, no. 15 (August 27, 1932).

24 Letter from acting surgeon general to Denney granting permission for patient Louie Chee to sell beer in his lunchroom, June 20, 1933, RG 90, Box 476, NACP.

25 Zachary Gussow, *Leprosy, Racism, and Public Health: Social Policy in Chronic Disease Control* (Boulder: Westview Press, 1989), 160.

26 "Is a Leprosarium a Place to Die?" *Sixty-Six Star*, August 15, 1933.

27 Michael Mizell-Nelson, "Treated as Lepers: The Patient-Led Reform Movement at the National Leprosarium, 1931–1946," *Louisiana History: The Journal of the Louisiana Historical Association*, 44, no. 3 (Summer 2003): 319.

28 Stein, *Alone No Longer*, 160.

Chapter 11: Search for a Cure

1 Tribute to Sister Hilary upon her retirement from Carville in 1960, by Father Alcuin Kammer, RG 10-2 Individual Sisters—Sr. Hilary Ross, DOC.

2 Stanley Stein, *Alone No Longer: The Story of a Man Who Refused to Be One of the Living Dead*, with Lawrence G. Blochman (New York: Funk and Wagnalls, 1963; repr., Star, 1974), 217.

3 Stein, *Alone No Longer*, 218.

4 O. E. Denney, "The National Leper Home (United States Marine Hospital), Carville, LA," *Public Health Reports*, 44, no. 52 (December 27, 1929): 3169–76.

5 O. E. Denney, "The National Leper Home (United States Marine Hospital), Carville, LA," *Public Health Reports*, 43, no. 14 (April 6, 1928), 810–17.

6 "My 37 Years at Carville," *Star*, 19, no. 6 (July–August 1960).

7 Sr. Hilary Ross, "Leprosarium, Carville, LA, 1894–1958," RG 11-2-2 Carville, LA—Hansen's Disease Center, DOC, 116.

8 "The Inside Story," *Star*, 13, no. 6 (February 1954).

9 Johnny Harmon, *King of the Microbes: The Autobiography of Johnny P. Harmon* (self-published, Carville, LA, produced by Franklin Press, 1995), 17.

10 Harmon, *King of the Microbes*, 27.

11 Entry dated December 30, 1935, in Daughters of Charity Annals, 1930–1939, vol. 4, 16769, NHDM.

12 From Koll's medical records at Carville. He gave this oral history on April 9, 1936.

13 New York *Daily News*, May 22, 1935.

14 U.S. Public Health Service letter to the Pullman Co. on procedures for transferring leprosy patients in their train cars, 1924, RG 90, Box 477, Folder L616 (1933–34), NACP.

15 Entries dated May 27–28, 1935, in Daughters of Charity Annals, 1930–1939, vol. 4, NHDM.

16 From Koll's oral history at Carville.

17 Julia Rivera Elwood, ed., *Known Simply to the Rest of the World as Carville, 100 Years, 1894–1994* (Washington, DC: U.S. Public Health Service, 1994), 46.

18 Elwood, *Known Simply*, 138.

19 Elwood, 178.

20 Tony Gould, *A Disease Apart: Leprosy in the Modern World* (New York: St. Martin's Press, 2005), 245.

21 "Death Ends Tragic Story of John Early, the Leper," *Asheville Citizen-Times*, March 1, 1938.

Chapter 12: Until Leprosy Do Us Part

1 Betty Martin, *Miracle at Carville*, edited by Evelyn Wells (New York: Doubleday, 1951), 70.

2 Conversation with former Carville social worker Bunny Harriman, Baton Rouge, LA, March 12, 2018.

3 Martin, *Miracle at Carville*, 86.

4 Martin, 80.

5 "A Need Is Filled," *Star*, 33, no. 3 (January–February 1974).

6 Stanley Stein, *Alone No Longer: The Story of a Man Who Refused to Be One of the Living Dead*, with Lawrence G. Blochman (New York: Funk and Wagnalls, 1963; repr., Star, 1974), 166.

7 Martin, *Miracle at Carville*, 113.

8 Martin, 114.

9 Inspection report from William Terriberry to U.S. surgeon general, January 10, 1935, RG 90, Box 479, Folder 1850-95 (1934–35), NACP.

10 Claire Manes, *Out of the Shadow of Leprosy* (Jackson: University Press of Mississippi, 2013), 93.

11 Author phone interview with Dolores Enriquez-Boehmer, April 9, 2018.

12 Marie Guerre's oral history, June 5, 1996, NHDM-21021.

13 From one of numerous interviews with NHDM curator Elizabeth Schexnyder, Carville, LA.

14 Johnny Harmon, *King of the Microbes: The Autobiography of Johnny P. Harmon* (self-published, Carville, LA, produced by Franklin Press, 1995), 71. Johnny's brother, Elmo, died at Carville in 1941.

15 Entry dated May 11, 1941, in Daughters of Charity Annals, 1940–1949, vol. 5, 16770, NHDM.

16 Marcia Gaudet, *Carville: Remembering Leprosy in America* (Jackson: University Press of Mississippi, 2004), 75; Harmon, *King of the Microbes*, 88.

17 Based on interviews with the patient and Carville social workers. This family preferred not to have the patient's name used.
18 Entry dated March 13, 1940, in Daughters of Charity Annals, 1940–1949.
19 Entry dated February 19, 1948, in Daughters of Charity Annals, 1940–1949.
20 Marie Guerre's oral history, NHDM.
21 Guerre, oral history.
22 Stein, *Alone No Longer*, 172.
23 Story told to author by former social workers at Carville.
24 Tony Gould, *A Disease Apart: Leprosy in the Modern World* (New York: St. Martin's Press, 2005), 245.
25 Stein, *Alone No Longer*, 171.
26 Martin, *Miracle at Carville*, 121.
27 Martin, 138.
28 Martin, 141–47.
29 Stein, *Alone No Longer*, 101.

Chapter 13: The Miracle

1   Betty Martin, *Miracle at Carville*, edited by Evelyn Wells (New York: Doubleday, 1951), 150.
2   Stanley Stein, *Alone No Longer: The Story of a Man Who Refused to Be One of the Living Dead*, with Lawrence G. Blochman (New York: Funk and Wagnalls, 1963; repr., Star, 1974), 216.
3   Stein, *Alone No Longer*, 189.
4   Stein, 193.
5   Stein, 207.
6   "Courage," *Star*, 1, no. 4 (December 1941).
7   Entry dated May 30, 1942, in Daughters of Charity Annals, 1940–1949, vol. 5, NHDM.
8   Entry dated March 19, 1940, in Daughters of Charity Annals, 1940–1949, vol. 5, NHDM.
9   Martin, *Miracle at Carville*, 182.
10 Sr. Hilary Ross, "Leprosarium, Carville, LA, 1894–1958," RG 11-2-2 Carville, LA—Hansen's Disease Center, DOC, 123.
11 Stein, *Alone No Longer*, 220–21.
12 Martin, *Miracle at Carville*, 197.
13 G. H. Faget et al., "The Promin Treatment of Leprosy: A Progress Report," *Public Health Reports*, 58, no. 48 (November 26, 1943): 1729–41.
14 E. Muir, "The South American Leprosy Conference," *Leprosy Review*, 18, no. 1 (1947).
15 Entry dated September 1, 1947, in Daughters of Charity Annals, 1940–1949, vol. 5, NHDM.
16 Stein, *Alone No Longer*, 222.

17 Entry dated May 1947 in Daughters of Charity Annals, 1940–1949, vol. 5, NHDM.

18 "How Can We Help," *Star*, 1, no. 5 (January 1942).

19 "Carville Patient Receives Citation from Treasury Department," *Star*, 2, no. 7 (March 1943).

20 Stein, *Alone No Longer*, 214.

21 Amy Fairchild, "Community and Confinement: The Evolving Experience of Isolation for Leprosy in Carville, Louisiana," *Public Health Reports*, 119 (May–June 2004), 365.

22 "Revise and Revoke!" *Star*, 2, no. 9 (May 1943).

23 "What the Patient Should Know about Hansen's Disease, IX, Rules and Regulations," *Star*, 2, no. 8 (April 1943).

24 "What the Patient Should Know about Hansen's Disease, VII," *Star*, 2, no. 6 (February 1943).

25 "What the Patient Should Know about Hansen's Disease, V, Treatment," *Star*, 2, no. 4 (December 1942).

26 "Hope Is Reborn Here" and "Editorial: Plain Talk," *Star*, 6, no. 1 (September 1946).

27 Marie Guerre's oral history, June 5, 1996, NHDM-21021.

28 Letter from Sister Zoe Schieswohl to Surgeon General Thomas Parran Jr., April 9, 1940, RG 90, Box 316, NACP.

29 "New World—New Hope—We Hope!" *Star*, 4, no. 2 (October 1944).

30 Stein, *Alone No Longer*, 231.

31 "Why Am I Not Free?" *Star*, 4, no. 11 (July 1945).

Chapter 14: Fighting for Freedom

1   Robert F. Rogers, *Destiny's Landfall: A History of Guam* (Honolulu: University of Hawaii Press, 1995), 136.

2   "Great Romance: The Major and His Lady," *Atlanta Constitution*, December 8, 1946.

3   "Major Hornbostel and Wife Arrive at U.S. Leprosarium," *Messenger-Inquirer* (Owensboro, KY), June 3, 1946.

4   Betty Martin, *Miracle at Carville*, edited by Evelyn Wells (New York: Doubleday, 1951), 251.

5   "Hero Seeks to Join Stricken Mate in Colony for Lepers," *San Francisco Examiner*, May 16, 1946.

6   Stanley Stein, *Alone No Longer: The Story of a Man Who Refused to Be One of the Living Dead*, with Lawrence G. Blochman (New York: Funk and Wagnalls, 1963; repr., Star, 1974), 249.

7   "Stigma More Dangerous Than Feebly Contagious Leprosy," *Montgomery Advertiser*, June 9, 1946.

8   "The Hornbostle [*sic*] Case," *Star*, 5, no. 10 (June 1946).

9   "Major Grateful Wife Has Leprosy instead of Cancer," *Alexandria Daily Town Talk*, June 3, 1946.

10 "As I See It," *Star*, 5, no. 11 (July 1946).

11 Stein, *Alone No Longer*, 249.

12 "Bill Would Allow Lepers to Vote," *Pensacola News Journal*, June 10, 1946.

13 Stein, *Alone No Longer*, 237.

14 Johnny Harmon, *King of the Microbes: The Autobiography of Johnny P. Harmon* (self-published, Carville, LA, produced by Franklin Press, 1995), 86.

15 "As I See It, After One Year," *Star*, 6, no. 10 (June 1947).

16 "The March of Educational Publicity," *Star*, 5, no. 12 (August 1946).

17 "Not Enough 'Life' in Carville for LIFE," *Star*, 6, no. 4 (December 1946).

18 "Helen Keller's Visit Brings Tonic Not Found in Materia Medica," *Star*, 4, no. 10 (June 1945).

19 Stein, *Alone No Longer*, 279.

20 Martin, *Miracle at Carville*, 271.

21 "Such Interesting Visitors," *Star*, 5, no. 12 (August 1946).

22 Cover illustration, *Star*, 6, no. 1 (September 1946).

23 "Patients Start on Initial Ride in Station Wagon," *Star*, 6, no. 4 (December 1946).

24 Martin, *Miracle at Carville*, 267.

25 Martin, 272.

26 Martin, 275–76.

27 "Holiday Highlights," *Star*, 6, no. 5 (January 1947).

Chapter 15: Not Bright Enough

1 Stanley Stein, *Alone No Longer: The Story of a Man Who Refused to Be One of the Living Dead*, with Lawrence G. Blochman (New York: Funk and Wagnalls, 1963; repr., Star, 1974), 231–33.

2 Stein, *Alone No Longer*, 238.

3 Stanley Stein's archives, 19733, NHDM.

4 Stein, *Alone No Longer*, 234–36; Madeleine Pierron Patrick, "The Secret People: Patriotism, the Press, and Civil Rights in the National Leprosarium" (master's thesis, University of Georgia, 2013), 61.

5 "A Summary of the Recommendations of the Advisory Committee on Leprosy in the United States," *Star*, 6, no. 5 (January 1947).

6 Entry dated January 1, 1948, in the Daughters of Charity Annals, 1940–1949, vol. 5, NHDM.

7 John Parascandola, "An Exile in My Own Country: The Confinement of Leprosy Patients at the United States National Leprosarium," *Medicina Nei Secoli (Journal of History of Medicine)*, 10, no. 1 (1998): 120–21.

8 Speech given by Sister Catherine at Carville, December 10, 1946, RG 10-2 Individual Sisters—Sr. Catherine Sullivan, DOC.

9 Editorial, *Star*, 7, nos. 7 and 8 (March–April 1948).

10 Betty Martin, *Miracle at Carville*, edited by Evelyn Wells (New York: Doubleday, 1951), 288–90.

11 "Progress in War against Darkness," *Star*, 6, no. 10 (June 1947).

12 Sr. Hilary Ross, "Leprosarium, Carville, LA, 1894–1958," RG 11-2-2 Carville, LA—Hansen's Disease Center, DOC, 112.

13 "Dr. Guy H. Faget 'Pioneer Sulfone Therapist' (1891 to 1947)," *Star*, 6, no. 12 (August 1947).

14 Stein, *Alone No Longer*, 243.

15 Stein, 278.

16 "Truth or Consequences," *Star*, 6, no. 7 (March 1947).

17 "A Rebuttal," *Star*, 6, no. 2 (October 1946).

18 Oral history of patient Nick Farrell, September 12, 1996, NHDM-21014.

19 "Actor Bergen Sets a Fine Example," *Tampa Times*, February 6, 1948.

20 Guerrero's life is the subject of a 2016 book by Ben Montgomery, *The Leper Spy: The Story of an Unlikely Hero of World War II*, published by Chicago Review Press. The use of the word *leper* in the title did not sit well with some former patients and Carville staff.

21 "First Impressions," *Star*, 7, no. 11 (August 1948).

22 "As I See It," *Star*, 8, no. 10 (June 1949).

23 NLM, PHSHHC, MS C 471, Box 11, Folder 8; Amy Fairchild, "Community and Confinement: The Evolving Experience of Isolation for Leprosy in Carville, Louisiana," *Public Health Reports*, 119 (May–June 2004): 366.

24 Based on oral history of patient who chose to remain anonymous, NHDM.

25 Hajime Sato and Janet E. Frantz, "Termination of the Leprosy Isolation Policy in the US and Japan: Science, Policy Changes, and the Garbage Can Model," *BMC International Health and Human Rights*, 5, no. 1 (March 16, 2005): 3.

Chapter 16: "It's Tallulah, Darling"

1 Stanley Stein, *Alone No Longer: The Story of a Man Who Refused to Be One of the Living Dead*, with Lawrence G. Blochman (New York: Funk and Wagnalls, 1963; repr., Star, 1974), 283.

2 Note from Stein to Tallulah Bankhead, August 6, 1950, Stanley Stein archives, 19878, NHDM.

3 Letter from Stein to Bankhead, August 7, 1950, 19878, NHDM.

4 Letter from Stein to Bankhead, September 19, 1950, 19878, NHDM.

5 Letter from Bankhead to Stein, undated (appears to have been her first letter to him, likely in the fall of 1950), 19878, NHDM.

6 Stein, *Alone No Longer*, 284.

7 Letter from Stein to José Ferrer, March 8, 1951, 19878, NHDM.

8 19878, NHDM.

9   "Life of Woman Leper a Fascinating Account," *Los Angeles Times*, November 26, 1950.

10 "Who Walk Alone—Modernized to Be Filmed," *Star*, 9, no. 4 (December 1949).

11 "Prespassing," *Star*, 9, no. 9 (May 1950).

12 Letter from Stein to Joy Lamont, May 15, 1951, 19878, NHDM.

13 Letter from Marlon Brando to Stein, undated (but prior to May 15, 1951), 19878, NHDM.

14 Letter from Stein to Brando, June 7, 1951, 19878, NHDM.

15 Stein, *Alone No Longer*, 231.

16 Stein, 266.

17 Dr. Frederick A. Johansen et al., "Promacetin in Treatment of Leprosy: Progress Report," *Public Health Reports*, 65, no. 7 (February 17, 1950).

18 Stein, *Alone No Longer*, 288.

19 Letter from Stein to "Everybody" at Carville, November 27, 1951, 19878, NHDM.

20 "Journey Proud," *Star*, 11, no. 5 (January 1952).

21 "Stanley Stein, Once Outcast as Leper, Gets Welcome Back," *Arizona Republic*, November 29, 1951.

22 Letter from Stein to Bankhead, December 31, 1951, 19878, NHDM.

23 "Victory over Hansen's Disease," *St. Louis Post-Dispatch*, January 6, 1952.

24 Stein, *Alone No Longer*, 294.

25 Stein, 297.

26 Stein, 301–2.

27 Entry dated June 18, 1953, in the Daughters of Charity Annals, 1950–1955, vol. 6, 16771, NHDM.

28 Stein, *Alone No Longer*, 305.

29 Raúl Necochea López, "Arresting Leprosy: Therapeutic Outcomes besides Cure," *American Journal of Public Health*, 108, no. 2 (February 2018): 196–202.

30 "There Have Been Some Changes Made," *Star*, 14, no. 4 (January 1955); Zachary Gussow, *Leprosy, Racism, and Public Health: Social Policy in Chronic Disease Control* (Boulder: Westview Press, 1989), 170.

31 Johnny Harmon, *King of the Microbes: The Autobiography of Johnny P. Harmon* (self-published, Carville, LA, produced by Franklin Press, 1995), 93.

32 Entry dated May 17, 1951, in the Daughters of Charity Annals, 1950–1955, vol. 6, NHDM.

33 Author interviews with Simeon Peterson, Baton Rouge, LA, May 23 and 26, 2016.

34 "V.I. Patients at Carville Sent Back to Islands," *Star*, 14, no. 6 (March 1955).

35 "The Sportsfolio, a Step Backwards," *State-Times* (Baton Rouge), August 6, 1956.

36 José P. Ramirez Jr., *Squint: My Journey with Leprosy* (Jackson: University Press of Mississippi, 2009), 118.

37 "Crisis at Carville, to Be Resolved, We Hope," *Star*, 16, no. 1 (September–October 1956).

38 "Carville in Future Hangs on Solution of Problems," *State-Times*, August, 25, 1956.

39 Tony Gould, *A Disease Apart: Leprosy in the Modern World* (New York: St. Martin's Press, 2005), 265.

Chapter 17: Human Touch

1 "Patients Appeal to Washington in Controversy at Carville," *State-Times* (Baton-Rouge), August 24, 1956.

2 "PHS Plan to Raze Cottages Raises Rumpus," *Star*, 16, no. 1 (September–October 1956). A transcript of the meeting can be found at the National Library of Medicine, PHSHHC, MS C 471, Box 12, Folder 10.

3 "VFW Auxiliary Is Asked to Assist Carville Patients," *State-Times*, September 11, 1956.

4 NLM, PHSHHC, MS C 471, Box 12, Folder 10.

5 "Passman Hints at Full Scale Probe at Carville," *State-Times*, August 24, 1956.

6 Stanley Stein, *Alone No Longer: The Story of a Man Who Refused to Be One of the Living Dead*, with Lawrence G. Blochman (New York: Funk and Wagnalls, 1963; repr., Star, 1974), 309.

7 "Congressman Passman's Visit—Real Turning Point," *Star*, 16, no. 1 (September–October 1956).

8 "Soviet-Type Prison Camp at Carville?" *Monroe Morning World*, August 26, 1956; Zachary Gussow, *Leprosy, Racism, and Public Health: Social Policy in Chronic Disease Control* (Boulder: Westview Press, 1989), 174.

9 "Carville Cottage Owners Question Administration," *Monroe Morning World*, August 29, 1956.

10 "Hospital Head Change Looms," *State-Times*, September 13, 1956.

11 "Crisis at Carville, to Be Resolved, We Hope," *Star*, 16, no. 1 (September–October 1956).

12 "New MOC Creates Favorable First Impression," *Star*, 16, no. 2 (November–December 1956).

13 "Golf Tourney Holds Spotlight Here," *Star*, 16, no. 2 (November–December 1956).

14 Betty Martin, *No One Must Ever Know* (New York: Doubleday, 1959), 82.

15 Martin, *No One Must Ever Know*, 231.

16 Stein, *Alone No Longer*, 329.

17 "Comments on Betty Martin's New Book," *Star*, 18, no. 5 (May–June 1959).

18 Martin, *No One Must Ever Know*, 202.

19 Ludwig G. Lederer, "The World of Science," *Hartford Courant*, August 23, 1959.
20 "Your Problems, by Ann Landers," *Press Democrat* (Santa Rosa, CA), February 8, 1959.
21 Author interview with Marguerite Kelly, Washington, DC, February 6, 2018.
22 "An Era Is Ended," *Star*, 18, no. 6 (July–August 1959).
23 Stein, Alone No Longer, 313.
24 "So Long, Bing—So Long, Old Pal," *Star*, 18, no. 6 (July–August 1959).

Chapter 18: An Era Ends

1 "French Nun-Scientist Visits Carville to Discuss Research on Hansen's Disease," *Star*, 14, no. 2 (October 1954).
2 Donald C. Geist, "Sister Marie Suzanne," *Records of the American Catholic Historical Society of Philadelphia*, 71, no. 3/4 (September, December 1960): 112–17.
3 "Death Takes Dedicated French Nun Scientist: Opinion Differs on Success of Her Research Work in HD," *Star*, 17, no. 3 (January–February 1958).
4 Stanley Stein, *Alone No Longer: The Story of a Man Who Refused to Be One of the Living Dead*, with Lawrence G. Blochman (New York: Funk and Wagnalls, 1963; repr., Star, 1974), 317.
5 Letter from Dr. George Fite to Sister Hilary Ross, May 8, 1958, RG 10-2 Individual Sisters—Sr. Hilary Ross, DOC.
6 Exchanges about tensions between Fite and Sr. Hilary in the spring of 1959 can be found at NLM, PHSHHC, MS C 471, Box 11, Folder 17.
7 Tribute to Sister Hilary upon her retirement by Father Alcuin Kammer, DOC.
8 Author interview with James Carville, New Orleans, LA, March 16, 2018.
9 "Rehabilitation Central Theme of Sixth Annual ALM-PHS Seminar," Star, 24, no. 5 (May–June 1965).
10 Margaret Brand also did groundbreaking work with leprosy patients. She determined that many were going blind because the bacilli damaged pain sensors on the surface of the eye and on the muscles that triggered blinking. Leprosy patients weren't blinking enough in response to pain, which meant their eyes were not being lubricated and were vulnerable to damage. She adopted a surgical procedure that had been developed for patients with Bell's palsy, connecting the muscle used for chewing to the eyelids. If patients regularly chewed gum they could avoid going blind.
11 Paul Brand and Philip Yancey, *Pain: The Gift Nobody Wants* (New York: HarperCollins, 1993), 160–65.
12 Stein, *Alone No Longer*, 324.

13 "Carville Bids Good-by to Valiant Editor: Four Chaplains Conduct Ecumenical Services," *Star*, 27, no. 3 (January–February 1968).

14 Brand and Yancey, *Pain*, 164–65.

15 *Star*, 27, no. 2 (November–December 1967). It's likely that Stein, a master at soliciting favorable comments from powerful figures, had a hand in crafting President Johnson's remarks about leprosy.

16 A three-patient board was set up and *The Star* would continue to publish long after Stein's death, under the sponsorship of the Forty and Eight veterans group. The circulation would grow to more than 84,000, in 150 countries. The paper was still being published as of 2020.

17 "Stanley Stein—He Lived to Serve Others," *Star*, 27, no. 3 (January–February 1968).

18 "Mailbag—The World Pays Tribute to Crusader," *Star*, 27, no. 3 (January–February 1968).

19 Cover, *Star*, 27, no. 3 (January–February 1968).

20 José P. Ramirez Jr., *Squint: My Journey with Leprosy* (Jackson: University Press of Mississippi, 2009). Details of Ramirez's experiences are based on his memoir and on author's phone interviews of Ramirez on May 20, 2016, and December 18, 2018, and numerous email exchanges.

21 Ramirez, *Squint*, 11–12.

22 Ramirez, 15.

Chapter 19: Discrimination

1 José P. Ramirez Jr., *Squint: My Journey with Leprosy* (Jackson: University Press of Mississippi, 2009), 58.

2 Oral history of Mary Ruth Daigle, March 21, 2002, NHDM-21009.

3 Oral history of Nancy Batista, May 29, 1996, NHDM-1989.

4 Report from Dr. Edgar B. Johnwick to the surgeon general, NLM, PHSHHC, MS C 471, Box 11, Folders 12–13.

5 "Mail Sterilization Ends," *Star*, 28, no. 3 (September–October 1968).

6 Conversation with former Carville social worker Bunny Harriman.

7 Ramirez, *Squint*, 80–81.

8 Author interviews with Simeon Peterson.

9 Ramirez, *Squint*, 63–64.

10 Ramirez, 62.

11 Ramirez, 120.

12 Ramirez, 122.

13 Ramirez, 103.

14 Ramirez, 116.

15 Ramirez, 116–17.

16 Ramirez, 124.

17 Recounted by Elizabeth Schexnyder, curator, NHDM.

18 Ramirez, *Squint*, 129–33.

19 "8 U.S. Hospitals Reported Closing," *New York Times*, December 19, 1970.
20 "Treatment Curbs Leprosy in 3 Months," *San Francisco Examiner*, February 17, 1970.
21 Paul Brand and Philip Yancey, *Pain: The Gift Nobody Wants* (New York: HarperCollins, 1993), 177–84; "Leprosy's Legacy," Washington Post, April 25, 1989.
22 Gordon Peterson, "Dateline: Florida Tech 1983: Secret History," Ad Astra (website), Florida Institute of Technology, August 14, 2018, https:// adastra.fit.edu/blog/campus/secret-history/rising-star-disney-comes-to -countdown-college-1983/.
23 "HD Transmitted to an Armadillo," *Star*, 30, no. 6 (July–August 1971).
24 "Armadillos: Their Capture and Care," *Star*, 31, no. 2 (November– December 1971).
25 "Research Grants Awarded," *Star*, 34, no. 6 (July–August 1975).
26 "Vietnam Girl, 9, Leprosy Patient," *Victoria Advocate*, August 22, 1977.
27 Author interview with Mien Pham, Gonzales, LA, March 21, 2018.

Chapter 20: Shutting Down

1 Other reports put the patient population at the time closer to three hundred.
2 Hajime Sato and Janet E. Frantz, "Termination of the Leprosy Isolation Policy in the US and Japan: Science, Policy Changes, and the Garbage Can Model," *BMC International Health and Human Rights*, 5, no. 1 (March 16, 2005).
3 "Congressional Hearing at NHDC," *Star*, 42, no. 1 (September–October 1982).
4 Zachary Gussow, *Leprosy, Racism, and Public Health: Social Policy in Chronic Disease Control* (Boulder: Westview Press, 1989), 196–97; "Plan Likely to Exempt Leprosy Research Center," *Shreveport Times*, September 4, 1982.
5 Centers for Disease Control and Prevention, *Morbidity and Mortality Weekly Report for June 18, 1982*. More background information can be found at https://www.hiv.gov.
6 "Mass. Neurosurgeon Suggests Quarantine for AIDS Carriers," *Boston Globe*, November 21, 1985.
7 "When Fear Conquers: A Doctor Learns about AIDS from Leprosy," *New York Times*, February 28, 1988.
8 "Talk of AIDS Quarantine Spreads Like a Disease," *Chicago Tribune*, November 12, 1985.
9 Ryan White and Ann Marie Cunningham, *Ryan White: My Own Story* (New York: Dial Books, 1991).
10 "Fury, Fear Mark Plan to Open Leprosy Clinic," *Muncie Evening Press*, April 24, 1987; "Tiny California Town Thwarts Plans for Leprosy Clinic," *Baltimore Sun*, June 22, 1987.
11 "Carville Patients Fear They Will Be Forced Out of Home," *Shreveport*

Times, March 12, 1999; "Residents Petition to Remain at Carville Facility," *The Advocate* (Baton Rouge), March 12, 1999; "First Annual International Day of Dignity and Respect," *Star*, 58, no. 1 (January–March 1999).

12 "Leprosy Center to Take 200 Ill U.S. Prisoners," *New York Times*, December 2, 1990.

13 For the best description of those years see Neil White, *In the Sanctuary of Outcasts* (New York: William Morrow/HarperCollins, 2009).

14 "Both Home and Prison, Leprosy Site May Shut," *New York Times*, June 23, 1998.

15 Marcia Gaudet, *Carville: Remembering Leprosy in America* (Jackson: University Press of Mississippi, 2004), 163.

16 "Ex-leprosy Patients Dreading Closure," *Daily Oklahoman*, March 27, 1999.

17 "The Only World They Know," *Newsweek*, March 28, 1999.

18 "We Have Suffered Too Long in Loneliness and in Fear," *Los Angeles Times*, December 14, 1997.

19 José P. Ramirez Jr., *Squint: My Journey with Leprosy* (Jackson: University Press of Mississippi, 2009), 184.

20 Vicki L. Pierre, "Living with Leprosy: Carville Patients in the Early Twentieth Century" (master's thesis, University of Minnesota, June 2012), 79.

21 Author interview with Dolores Enriquez-Boehmer by phone, April 9, 2018.

22 "Confined by Leprosy, but Open to the World: Remembering 'Ambassador' Mr. Pete," by author, NPR News, December 28, 2017.

23 Author interview with Linda Williams by phone, April 13, 2018.

24 Author interview with Claire Manes, Lafayette, LA, March 15, 2018.

25 Gaudet, *Carville*, 179.

26 Claire Manes, *Out of the Shadow of Leprosy* (Jackson: University Press of Mississippi, 2013), 143–44.

27 Author phone interview with Gina DeRose Bell, May 2, 2018.

28 "New Jersey Accepts Rights for People in Quarantine to End Ebola Suit," *New York Times*, July 27, 2017.

Chapter 21: Lessons Not Learned

1 Based on statistics from the Centers for Disease Control and Prevention and the World Health Organization, including WHO's *Weekly Epidemiological Record*, no. 35 (September 2, 2016).

2 Based on author's numerous interviews with current and former employees of the National Hansen's Disease Program, including director Dr. David Scollard.

3 "Leprosy Worries Remain for Some Jurupa Valley Parents," *Press-Enterprise*, September 24, 2016.

4 Author interview with Francisco Sanchez, Carville, LA, May 25, 2016.

5 NPR News, interview on *Weekend Edition Sunday*, May 12, 2019.

6 "Leprosy, a Synonym for a Stigma, Returns," *New York Times*, February 18, 2003.

7 Vicki L. Pierre, "Living with Leprosy: Carville Patients in the Early Twentieth Century" (master's thesis, University of Minnesota, June 2012), 80–82; "Truth, Fiction and Lou Dobbs," *New York Times*, May 30, 2007.

8 "Trump's Arguments for Necessity of Border Wall Have Already Been Broadly Debunked," *Washington Post*, December 11, 2018.

9 Author interview with Daniel Cabrera, Baton Rouge, LA, May 24, 2016.

10 Author interview with Ramón Cabrera, Carville, LA, March 27, 2018.

Selected Bibliography

ARCHIVES

Daughters of Charity Archives, Province of St. Louise, Emmitsburg, MD
(Carville, LA—National Hansen's Disease Center Collection)

Louisiana State University Libraries, Baton Rouge, LA (Louisiana and
Lower Mississippi Valley Collections—Louisiana Leper Home Records)

National Library of Medicine, Bethesda, MD (Public Health Service
Hospitals Historical Collection)

National Archives and Records Administration, College Park, MD (Public
Health Service records)

National Hansen's Disease Museum, Carville, LA

Numerous newspaper and publication archives, including *The Star*, the
Times-Picayune, *The Advocate*, and *Public Health Reports*

BOOKS

Arnold, James R. *The Moro War: How America Battled a Muslim Insurgency in
the Philippine Jungle, 1902–1913*. New York: Bloomsbury Press, 2011.

Brand, Paul, and Philip Yancey. *Pain: The Gift Nobody Wants*. New York:
HarperCollins, 1993.

Brody, Saul Nathaniel. *The Disease of the Soul: Leprosy in Medieval Literature*.
Ithaca and London: Cornell University Press, 1974.

Burgess, Perry. *Who Walk Alone: A Man's Life with Leprosy and the Sanctuary of
Sorrow*. New York: Henry Holt, 1940.

Elwood, Julia, ed. *With Love in Their Hearts: The Daughters of Charity of St. Vincent de Paul, 1896–1996.* Washington, DC: U.S. Public Health Service, 1996.

——. *Known Simply to the Rest of the World as Carville . . . 100 Years, 1894–1994.* Washington, DC: U.S. Public Health Service, 1994.

Gaudet, Marcia. *Carville: Remembering Leprosy in America.* Jackson: University Press of Mississippi, 2004.

Gould, Tony. *A Disease Apart: Leprosy in the Modern World.* New York: St. Martin's Press, 2005.

Gussow, Zachary. *Leprosy, Racism, and Public Health: Social Policy in Chronic Disease Control.* Boulder: Westview Press, 1989.

Harmon, Johnny P. *King of the Microbes: The Autobiography of Johnny P. Harmon.* Self-published, Carville, LA, produced by Franklin Press, 1995. (In 2019, Anne Harmon Brett edited and self-published an adaptation of her father's memoir, with additional notes, called *The Disease: One Man's Journey through a Life with Leprosy.*)

Heiser, Victor. *An American Doctor's Odyssey: Adventures in Forty-Five Countries.* New York: W. W. Norton, 1936.

Kendall, John Smith. *History of New Orleans.* Chicago and New York: Lewis Publishing Company, 1922.

Manes, Claire. *Out of the Shadow of Leprosy: The Carville Letters and Stories of the Landry Family.* Jackson: University Press of Mississippi, 2013.

Martin, Betty. *Miracle at Carville.* Edited by Evelyn Wells. New York: Doubleday, 1951.

——. *No One Must Ever Know.* New York: Doubleday, 1959.

Moran, Michelle T. *Colonizing Leprosy: Imperialism and the Politics of Public Health in the United States.* Chapel Hill: University of North Carolina Press, 2007.

Oshinsky, David M. *Polio: An American Story.* New York: Oxford University Press, 2005.

Parascandola, John. *Sex, Sin and Science: A History of Syphilis in America.* Westport, CT: Praeger, 2008.

Ramirez, José P., Jr. *Squint: My Journey with Leprosy.* Jackson: University Press of Mississippi, 2009.

Sontag, Susan. *Illness as Metaphor.* New York: Farrar, Straus and Giroux, 1978.

Stein, Stanley. *Alone No Longer: The Story of a Man Who Refused to Be One of the Living Dead.* With Lawrence G. Blochman. New York: Funk and Wagnalls, 1963. Reprinted in 1974 by *The Star.*

Tayman, John. *The Colony: The Harrowing True Story of the Exiles of Molokai.* New York: Scribner, 2006.

Wallace, Lew. *Ben-Hur: A Tale of the Christ*. Blacksburg, VA: Wilder Publications, 2011. First published 1880 by Harper & Brothers (New York).

White, Neil. *In the Sanctuary of Outcasts*. New York: William Morrow/Harper Collins, 2009.

DOCUMENTARY FILMS

Harrison, Laura, and John Anderson, directors. *Secret People: The Naked Face of Leprosy in America*. 1999.

Wilhelm, John, director, writer, and producer, and Sally Squires, writer and producer. *Triumph at Carville: A Tale of Leprosy in America*. 2005. The Wilhelm Group. Distributed by PBS Home Video.

Index